"If you are facing an oropharyngeal can's
book will give you an idea c |"
and will give you hope that
you can come out the other
to the fullest, just as John ha

"No Quit in Me" is an enlightening raw look into the daily routine of dealing with head and neck cancer. A definite "must read" for anyone dealing with this type of cancer."

Gerry Simpson - mountain biker
also treated for head and neck cancer

"WOW! John Kuby's book captures exactly the thoughts, feelings and experiences I went through four years ago with the same cancer - same location on my tongue, same protocol and same great results! I wish I could have read this to know what to expect. It would have been so helpful. Others will benefit from this for sure."

Lee Sowell - Tongue cancer
survivor/businessman/skier/biker

"John's raw and authentic account of his tongue cancer experience is told with humour and compassion. Health care providers will be recommending this book as an inspiration for true patient engagement."

Lynda Brown - CEO, Curatio Networks, Inc.

"Anyone treating patients with this type of cancer, in any capacity, should consider this as a mandatory reference for their patients. Quite simply, oropharyngeal and tongue cancer patients and their caregivers need to read this book."

Dr. Ian Thornton - DDS, MSc, Dip Prostho. FRCD

"There is an honesty and a vulnerability that is rare, particularly among men, who are actively discouraged from being vulnerable in our culture, especially men of his generation and older. John has broken free of that. His writing is significant and refreshing."

Donaleen Saul - "No Quit in Me" book editor
Author of "Did You Know that I Would Miss You?"

"I found the book to be fantastic, it really painted a vivid picture of what John went through. It will be an excellent resource for those going into a cancer battle and for the caregivers along for the wild ride."

Simon Conde – Chiropractor

"No Quit in Me" offers authentic, relatable companionship for patients and their support people."

Shannon Moise - mountain biker/skier

"When my husband was diagnosed with throat cancer our oncologist suggested we check out John Kuby's blog. What a godsend! The doctors tell you the treatment will bring you to your knees. But when you can no longer eat, speak, or lift yourself from the couch, you desperately want to know how long each difficult phase will last. Thanks to John story, we had a guide through the wilderness of throat cancer treatment and survival. Although everyone's journey is slightly different, it's comforting to follow someone who has been there and come out the other end."

Catherine Szabo - wife of a throat cancer survivor

"This is a must-read for anyone fighting head or neck cancer, along with their family members and caregivers. While it's an unvarnished look at what to expect, Kuby's optimism through-out provides the reader with much-needed hope."

John Brockenbrough
- Creative Director/Brand Strategy Consultant

"I found myself constantly saying, "Yes!", "Good for you!" and "That's right!" as I read it. I felt like I had joined John in the winners circle when the book was finished."

Ben Prins – President,
Active Playground Equipment, Ltd.

"I never would have thought that a book that describes "mucus" so many times, could be so engaging and thought-provoking. What a remarkably open and honest account of a battle with cancer, chemo, and radiation! By chronicling his fight and writing with wry wit along way, John Kuby is sure to both help and entertain a wide variety of readers who face health struggles. "No Quit in Me" has inspired me to "Harden the F__k up", no matter what challenges I may face in my future!"

Paul Shore - Technology Consultant, and
Author of "Uncorked: My Year in Provence"

"No Quit in me is a raw and authentic glimpse into John's journey through tongue cancer and life after. He shares the power of his "no quit" mindset and provides relatable lessons to build your own resiliency when life gets painful. John's passion for physical fitness, gratefulness towards his family and friends, and his ability to be emotionally vulnerable is truly inspirational."

Jen Taubensee - Occupational Therapist.

"As a tongue cancer survivor, I support your book and you John. While sometimes unsettling, "No Quit in Me" is a fascinating and important guide for anyone facing this disease, or for loved ones trying to cope with someone who is. While our shared paths have similar trajectories in the arena of trauma both physically and mentally, your journey is uniquely yours. Each of us have our own challenges. The woman who mentored me through the early part of my own journey who used to say, "You don't know what you don't know." This is especially true with cancer. Your book goes a long way to shedding some light on what we don't know and should be read by anyone facing down the barrel of this gun."

Gary Harvey - Fellow tongue cancer survivor

"I can't imagine being closer to the experience without having tongue cancer myself."

Dr. Michael Henry - Dean, School of Business
& Economics, Thompson Rivers University

"John's writing is fluid and compelling, drawing the reader into the immediacy and uncertainty of living day to day with and through this illness. A must read."

Jane Hewes - Faculty of Education and
Social Work, Thompson Rivers University

"When reading this story, this documentation of a journey, you will laugh, you will cry, you will be informed, but most importantly, you will understand what the title "No Quit in Me" really means!"

John Tansowny and Peggy Arbeau
Family friends of John and Linda

"I recommend this book to anyone looking to understand what the of the experience of tongue cancer can be like, and to those looking for hope and inspiration for getting through their own challenging times."

Dr. J. Lauren Johnson - Registered Psychologist

NO QUIT IN ME

NO QUIT IN ME

MY WILD RIDE WITH TONGUE CANCER

BY JOHN KUBY

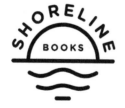

Cover and Book Design by JP King
Author Photograph by Michael Kuby

Although the author and publisher have made every effort to ensure the accuracy and completeness of information contained in this book, we assume no responsibility for errors, inaccuracies, omissions, or any inconsistency herein. Any slights of people, places, or organizations are unintentional.

This book is not intended as a substitute for appropriate medical intervention. Readers should consult a qualified medical professional with respect to any symptoms that may require diagnosis or medical attention.

For more information, please contact johnkuby@gmail.com
www.noquitinme.ca

ISBN 978-1-9993801-1-3 (paperback)

To my wife, Linda Diane Rasmussen

My true companion

FOREWORD

—

A LIFE COACH'S PERSPECTIVE

When John decided to blog and to share his cancer experience with his friends and colleagues, I was interested in reading what he had to say and in offering my help to him and to his wife, Linda. I thought I was doing him a favour by following him, but what I found out was that I was receiving one of the greatest gifts one human being can ever give to another – his innermost thoughts, feelings, and experiences. The real and unabridged version of himself.

Week by week, month by month, I not only learned about what a tongue cancer patient contends with, but I also learned about perseverance, about strength, about community, about support, and about what it felt like to be going through all the experiences that John and Linda were facing. John was a researcher, a mentor, a model, an inspiration, and a leader to all of us who followed his blog. I saw his spirit soar and sink and soar again. Through his words, I watched him prevail over incredibly difficult circumstances and come out the victor, because he faced the fear and did whatever it took to triumph over what seemed like impossible challenges. Even if his body never fully recovers, although I think with his tenacity it will, he will be the winner because he did not and does not let the "small stuff" of cancer get in the way of creating the life he wants and loves to live.

John thinks this book is about supporting individuals with tongue cancer, and indeed it is, but I think it is also about creating the life we want and finding a way to make it happen. John's spirit, his vision, his willingness to be vulnerable, and his generosity in sharing every step of his journey are remarkable. As his readers, we have found a true champion of the human spirit and a pathway for overcoming whatever lies ahead for us.

Anne Ryan
Relationship Coach

—

AN ONCOLOGIST'S PERSPECTIVE

Oropharyngeal cancer has become the most common head and neck cancer that we see in our clinic. It, unfortunately, affects people whom you wouldn't expect to get a cancer that used to be caused by smoking and excessive drinking. We are now seeing an epidemic of young, healthy people, just like John, diagnosed with this devastating illness.

There is no easy treatment for head and neck cancer. Surgery can be extremely morbid. Radiation and chemotherapy have side effects that can last a lifetime. Patients agonize over what treatment is best for them. John was one of them. As a radiation oncologist, I, along with my medical oncology and surgical colleagues, try to give patients like John the information they need to make well-informed decisions.

There is, however, a lack of information on the experience through the patient's eyes. John's blog, and now this book, "No

Quit in Me", attempts to capture this vital piece of the puzzle that will help new patients anticipate some of what they are heading into.

I've followed John's blog since its inception and have recommended it to my patients. He's gone through an incredible journey, from his diagnosis, through his treatment, to the long-term effects of the cancer and treatment on his body, which he is now dealing with. He's had ups and downs, both physically and mentally. His experience will not be the same as yours, but it will give you and your family an idea of what to expect, of what is "normal." Most importantly, it will give you hope that, despite all the challenges of cancer, you can come out the other side and continue to live your life to the fullest, just like John.

Dr. Brock Debenham, Radiation Oncologist
Cross Cancer Institute; Edmonton, Alberta

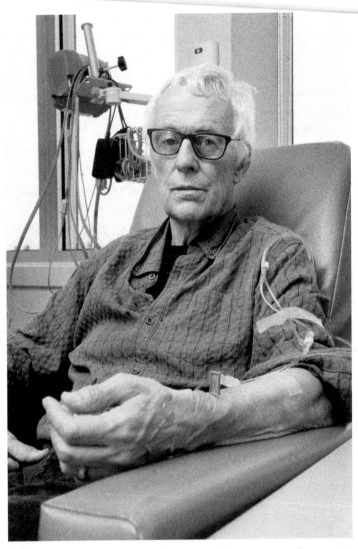

To view a photo essay of John's Cancer experience please visit
www.michaelkuby.com or www.noquitinme.ca

A full timeline of events and experiences, which compliment each chapter, is provided at the end of the book.

CONTENTS

INTRODUCTION

—

CAPTURING CANCER IN WORDS

"We tell ourselves stories in order to live." Joan Didion

I initially told my tongue cancer story in a blog called "Cancer, but No Quit in Me." I wanted to share how it felt to discover that I had cancer, and to follow my treatment and recovery experiences through to the end. I wasn't sure what the end would be. There was a lot of fear in the beginning.

I'm writing this introduction a year after my diagnosis and after writing more than 80 blogs about my experience. I chose *No Quit in Me* as my title because I thought it would offer hope and inspiration for my readers. I also chose it for me; I needed to remind myself that there really is no quit in me. Sometimes I had to fake my no quit in me attitude with those who supported me, but faking it 'til I made it ended up working for me. I fooled myself into believing I could do this.

A month before I was diagnosed with cancer, I heard a guest on CBC radio talk about journaling being therapeutic. She said that people who journaled about difficult or painful events seemed to heal more quickly and that cancer patients tended to be among them. I remember saying to myself at the time, "If I ever get cancer, I'm going to journal." Little did I know how prophetic that statement would be.

Because I'm a show-off kind of guy who's comfortable disclosing my feelings and communicating my experiences, good or bad, it was natural for me to turn my journal into a blog. In fact, I couldn't wait to get it set up on-line, so I could start sharing what I was going through. My wife, Linda, will tell you that I was super impatient, insisting that she set it up for me – right now! I wanted to capture my exact feelings as they arose. I wanted to write about everything that was happening and to get it out there.

What I wasn't able to predict was how beneficial the blog would be. I think people were surprised, and so was I, at how effective my writing was at expressing what I was going through. It was gratifying to have struck a chord with up to 350 readers a day, many of whom had faced or were facing something similar – or worse. Knowing that I had people following my story motivated me to continue to write, and to write as well as I could.

The blog also made me feel better about myself and my capacity to deal with my challenges. When dealing with the effects of chemotherapy and recovery from radiation, you need to gather strength from wherever you can get it. Writing my story was therapeutic. Having a caring audience gave me strength and encouragement.

That's what this story is about: recovery, strength, endurance, and hope.

I'm not an expert on cancer, or even tongue cancer. I'm only an expert on my own experience – from the shock of my initial diagnosis of oropharyngeal cancer to where I am today. I no longer have cancer and I've recovered, but I'm still discovering and dealing with a "new normal" for my health and for my life.

What I find surprising is that I no longer have a clear memory of what I experienced during the treatment and initial recovery period. It's all a blur to me now. Good thing I had it all captured in my blogs. Rereading them to incorporate them into my book made me realize, Wow! Cancer is tough shit! Radiation recovery is tough shit! One of the lessons I've learned is that no matter how excruciating things may feel in the moment, it is always true that "This too shall pass." These are hard words to believe when you're lying in bed in the middle of the night, wide awake, exhausted, fixating on the thick phlegm build-up at the top of your throat. Especially if you're convinced that the phlegm will choke you if you fall asleep.

The words, "This too shall pass" reminded me of my dad's response whenever us kids would whine and complain about our troubles. He would often say, "Ya, it goes on like that for a while... (pause for effect) ... and then it gets worse!"

Worse? How helpful was that message, which is still with me decades later? I think the fear that it's all going to get worse is what makes cancer even scarier than it already is. Cancer just is a scary thing. So are radiation and chemotherapy. The scariness doesn't need embellishing.

I started to take seriously the idea of turning the blog into a book when my oncologist told me he was sending his new cancer patients to read it. After meeting with a couple of his patients and learning that they were hungry for the information I was providing, I started to think that this book might be useful for all tongue cancer patients and their caregivers. I also had professional caregivers saying that I was a textbook example of how they wanted patients to deal with cancer and radiation/chemotherapy recovery, and with recovery in general.

Yes, I handled my cancer experience in a way that I'm proud of, but it wouldn't have happened without a lot of support. For that I am truly thankful. Rereading my blog posts through the course of writing this book made me realize that I had a lot of help. Thankfulness had to become one of the themes of my recovery story.

I got a ton of support from my wife, my family, my friends, many acquaintances and business associates, all of the professionals at the hospitals I visited over the last year and a half, and all of the people reading and commenting on my blog. I asked everyone for help and I got it. I got love and attention, right when I needed it most. Sure, I was blessed, but my guess is that everyone who goes through shit like this will get the help they need if they ask for it, if they're open to accepting it, and if they're appreciative upon receiving it.

Another of the themes in the book is my awareness of how important physical activity is. I am going into my seventies and still mountain biking and snowboarding. I also do yoga and resistance training. All my life I have been on again off again active at something, mostly on, mostly at hockey. I started biking and snowboarding in my late 40's and early 50's. My riding buddies all agree that the only reason we are still riding in our 60's is because unlike most men our age we just didn't ever quit. There are many good reasons guys slow down and quit; careers, wives, kids, houses, drinking, weight gain, decline in ability, injury and a lack of support and encouragement. We managed to overcome each of these and we are still active. We would not let ourselves quit.

When I was recovering I was bound and determined to get back the joy and satisfaction I feel when I am active. That gave me the motivation and incentive to hang in there and do all the right things to aid and speed up my recovery. And now I am out riding my bike and my board. Not yet as strong as I was but I will get there. No quit.

One of the many benefits I got from writing the blog was that it provided a lot of "me time." Gary Harvey, also a tongue cancer survivor and one of my mentors, told me not to worry about being selfish during recovery. "Recovery time is 'me time,'" he said. "Take it. It's your time to take care of yourself." I'm thankful for that piece of advice. I spent a big part of my "me time" writing blog posts and responding to readers' comments. The writing was therapeutic and cathartic; putting it in blog form connected me to a much larger caregiver community. I got a lot of helpful advice and encouragement from my readers, especially from those who had been through their own cancer experiences. According to the Canadian Cancer Society, almost 45% of women and 49% of men will be diagnosed with cancer at some point in their lives.

As I went through my cancer adventure, I was surprised to discover just how many of my friends had been affected by cancer. I'm humbled to realize that I'd been too busy with the various dramas of my own life to acknowledge or even be aware of their cancer-related issues. Having gone through what I've gone through, I'm determined to be more aware and to have much more compassion for cancer victims from now on.

— To view a photo essay of John's cancer experience please visit www.michaelkuby.com or www.noquitinme.ca

LESSONS LEARNED: INTRODUCTION CAPTURING CANCER IN WORDS

- Journaling engages your healing muscle. Write it down.
- Don't panic. This too shall pass.
- Share your experiences with others, without whining. Help them care about you.
- Ask for help.
- Be thankful for the support.
- Do your part to make yourself stronger and healthier.
- Make it your goal to heal and get back to normal.
- Be aware that you are not the only one with troubles.

LINDA'S CAREGIVER NOTES:

Unfortunately, I did not take the time to write about what was happening to me while supporting John through his illness, and so what you are reading now are my recollections as his primary caregiver during his treatment and recovery.

Although I had parented two of my own children and two stepchildren, I had never had to look after someone with a serious illness who needed months of care. The funny thing is that in my late twenties I wanted to be a nurse, but after a nine-week career counselling program, I discovered that I lacked a number of the key attributes of a good nurse – attention to detail, organizational ability, discipline, and emotional stability!

More importantly, I didn't want to work with sick people; I was far more interested in keeping people healthy. In the end, I worked in health promotion and policy development. I worked with nurses, but I was not a nurse.

Also, I'm not so sure that I have enough empathy to be a nurse. When John took up mountain biking in his 50s, his class was taken by helicopter to the top of a mountain which they were to ride down. I told him that we had disability insurance but no life insurance, so if he found himself hurling down the mountain out of control, he should go hard. We couldn't afford him being disabled!

Supporting John through his illness was a challenge for both of us. It changed our roles and our relationship. This kind of responsibility can be all-encompassing and, like many women, I didn't know where to draw the line. There was always more that I could or should do.

I needed "me time" too, but I found it hard to reach out for help. I found that physical activity reduced my stress and gave me time away from all the things that I felt I "had" to do. Working on the exercise machines at Curves was mindless and I didn't need to talk to anyone. It took me a long time before I could share with the women at Curves what I was going through.

DISCOVERY:

OH SHIT,
I HAVE CANCER!

DID SHE JUST TELL ME
I HAVE CANCER?

Just after Christmas, 2015, I was having a little trouble hearing and went in to see my doctor to have wax cleared from my ears. He cleared out some wax but also told me the hearing problem was from inflammation that was congesting my nasal passages and prescribed a nasal spray.

The nasal spray did nothing. The congestion just persisted. So I went back to the doctor and he prescribed an antibiotic. Unfortunately, that did nothing either. My throat even started to develop some hoarseness and irritation.

A month later, I was back seeing my doctor again, and he identified inflamed lymph nodes in my neck. No biggie, I thought. Inflamed lymph nodes happen all the time, don't they? My doctor didn't seem worried. I jokingly suggested that it must be cancer since there seemed to be no other explanation for the perniciousness of this cold, or whatever it was. We chuckled. Then the doctor ordered some blood work. Didn't we already do that? What would more blood work tell us?

I didn't hear about any blood work results for what seemed like a long time, so I called the clinic. My doctor was on a brief holiday; I bugged them into letting me see the back-up doctor. She felt the lymph nodes and told me I needed to get an ultrasound. She got me in pretty quick.

The imaging must have shown something, because a radiologist came in to speak with me immediately. He said that the ultrasound was inconclusive, and I would probably need a CT scan (computer-processed combinations of many x-ray measurements). Very calm, no panic. The lymph nodes were swollen. That happens. But these were an irregular shape, so there was some concern. He was careful not to say concern about what. I guess they don't mention cancer if they don't have to. It spooks people. I never had any inkling that it was cancer. I'm a healthy guy. I exercise a lot. I eat well. I take care of myself. I'm not the kind of guy who gets cancer.

That was in the morning. That afternoon the back-up doctor left me a message with a cell number to call her at home that night about the results. I called her that evening. She was very caring and concerned, but there was no panic. I thought she was just being thorough and kind. She reiterated what the other doctor had said about the irregular shape of the lymph nodes, and said that they had booked me in for a CT scan next week. There was a discussion about having to be sure of this or that, and an ever-so-vague mention that there could be cancer.

I told her that I was going on a snowboarding trip and wouldn't be back for six days. We agreed that she would try to get me in for the scan after my return. As she finished the call, she quietly said that she was sorry that I had to find out about this over the phone. "This?" I thought to myself. "What's 'this?'"

As I hung up, I realized that "this" must be cancer.

Did she just tell me I have cancer? Shit!

Linda had been in the kitchen listening to the call. When I hung up, she gave me a huge hug and said, "Sweetie, you'll be OK. We'll get through this." After that, we didn't talk or think about it much. Did I really have cancer? Nah. Not me.

The CT scan happened at noon, the day after I got back from my snowboarding trip, which was fantastic. A couple of hours later, the clinic booked me in to see Dr. Bruchette, my family doctor. Linda came with me. When Dr. Bruchette entered the room he was very direct, as he always is. He quickly and clearly told me it was cancer. Cancer on the back of my tongue. It wouldn't kill me. It could probably be removed with surgery. With a great deal of sympathy and concern, he said, "This is an ugly place to have cancer. It affects how you talk and how you eat, so it has big impacts on every aspect of your life. Recovery is going to be long and hard."

Apart from the radiation I would need after surgery, there would be other recovery issues. If the saliva glands are affected, I could have dry mouth, and swallowing might be painful. I might have to have my tongue rebuilt in order to be able to talk. As he said, "This is not a good cancer." The doctor spoke of a famous football player, Jim Kelly, bravely fighting his tongue cancer for five years, but eventually recovering.

Five years of recovery? Really?

But, I'm not likely to die from it. I guess that's the good news.

He said the next step was to find out if it has spread. That could be dangerous depending on where it has spread to. Also, they would need to determine more about the type of cancer and the stage. In addition, he told me that he had referred me to a surgeon at the University of Alberta Hospital who is "the best." Dr. Jeffrey Harris is the doctor he would want if he had this cancer. There was some comfort in knowing that.

Linda was with me for that discussion. We couldn't say it out loud, but this was worse than we thought. But we'd get through it. I think we were more worried about this screwing up our holiday plans than we were about cancer. It's hard for the reality of the pain and suffering part of cancer to sink in. We ended our discussion with another big hug, and a reassuring, "We'll get through this, Sweetie," from Linda.

We looked up our doctor's credentials on the internet and they were impeccable.

We also looked up throat cancer. It's ugly. Recovery is difficult, and it takes a long time.

When it's cancer, the medical system must work more quickly. That same afternoon, we were at the University of Alberta Hospital talking to a head and neck surgeon to do a "work up," whatever that means. The hand-offs from doctor to doctor were tricky. They didn't know what we knew or didn't know, so they were very careful. The next doctor I spoke to asked us if we knew why we were there and I said, "I'm in a cancer ward. I'm talking to a cancer surgeon, I think I have cancer." He laughed.

The tumor is way back in my throat, at the base of my tongue. He couldn't see it through my mouth, so he put a scope through my nostril to get a look at it. It's about six centimeters in diameter. Pretty big, according to him.

Before they know what my treatment schedule will be, they'll need a PET (Positron Emission Tomography) scan, which uses a form of radioactive sugar to create images of body function and metabolism. They'll also need a biopsy. That should take a couple of weeks. When the surgery takes place is determined by the results and by availability.

Then we met a nurse who said she was going to be my contact at that office. She seemed very efficient, reassuring and helpful. She gave me her phone number and email address. I dubbed her my "cancer coach." Coach Lisa. She seemed OK with that.

That was Friday. A little stunned by the news, we went out for supper at an upscale restaurant. I played the sympathy card with the waiter and was given a free dessert. Linda was a bit embarrassed.

On Monday, I got a call booking me for the PET Scan for the upcoming Thursday.

Not sure when the biopsy will happen. What is a biopsy?

On Monday morning, I had a meeting with all 12 staff of my company, PlayWorks, which sells playground equipment to schools and communities, and told them all about the cancer diagnosis. They were shocked, of course, and promised to take care of the business while I took care of my health. As I spoke, I noticed that my voice was hoarse and I had some trouble talking. My throat was starting to hurt.

Now I'm worried. I don't like pain. The prospect of suffering is starting to make this whole cancer thing seem much more real.

I hope it doesn't get too real too fast.

IT'S STARTING TO SINK IN

I have cancer. It's not fair. Of course, it's not fair.

Am I afraid? Of course, I am.

It is going to be painful, frustrating, and inconvenient, but I will survive.

And I will recover and heal quickly.

How do I know? I'd heard on CBC radio that people who journal about their illnesses recover faster. I believe in CBC radio, so I'm going to journal about my experience.

How do I know I'll survive? Because it's tongue cancer. I don't think tongue cancer kills people. But it could, I guess. It is cancer after all, so I am justified in feeling apprehensive.

I'm afraid of what it's going to take to survive. What will I have to endure? My doctor made it very clear that this would be an ugly process. I could have trouble swallowing. I could lose a lot of strength and vitality. I could lose my saliva glands and have dry mouth all the time. I may even have to learn to talk again. And it will be painful

It will be hard, but I will endure because there is no quit in me. I will weaken, but I will not give up. I will do whatever it takes. I'm 68 years old. I've endured a lot of shit in my life and I'm a better person for every challenge I've ever faced. I've endured two divorces, two brushes with business bankruptcy, and some serious health challenges, including infectious hepatitis A and ulcerative colitis. I'd always thought that "shit like that" belonged in the past and that there would be clear sailing ahead once I got past it. But I guess there's always another pile of shit coming. The more piles of shit you sail through, the more faith you have that the next pile won't stop you.

As my mountain biking friends, the F'n Riders, and my snowboarding buddies, the Pow-Pow Crushers, have all noticed, I fall a lot, but I always get up from a fall and carry on. I fall because I'm always pushing the boundaries of my fears and abilities; that's where the fun in life is.

And I will thrive because I have a strong support network that's here to help me when I fall. Already I've received a sincere outpouring of concern from everyone who knows about my cancer. My number one support person, my wife Linda, isn't panicking. She continues to be the rock I can lean on.

Her twin sister, Lorna, has recently been hospitalized with a heart issue, so Linda has more than me to worry about. Her sympathy muscles will be strained, but I've always been able to count on her and I'm sure she will guide me through this. No pressure, Linda!

Linda, if I forget to mention you in this book as often as you deserve, it's not because I don't love and appreciate you. It's because you're like breathing to me. I rarely stop to appreciate the fact that I'm breathing.

It's been particularly gratifying to get emails, phone calls and hugs from the 24 guys with whom I'd gone snowboarding just before getting the cancer diagnosis. They'd known I was coughing up blood the last night we were together, so they were the first to be concerned. I was almost euphoric reading their messages. As Linda said, it's been like hearing what people say about you at your funeral without having to die first. The expressions of praise and admiration I got from these young guys all landed in the right place.

Compliments don't have to be a 100% true. They just need a believable amount of truth to work their magic.

I've had lots of great advice, wisdom, and offers of help from everyone who knows about my cancer. I'm now coming to think of you all as my support team. My support buddies. The term, "buddy," comes from my new snowboarding friend, Ryan deMilliano. He reminded me of what our cat ski guide had told us. "In the back country we're all buddies. When you see someone go down, he's your buddy. You stop and see if he's OK. You see that he gets up."

My snowboarder buddies also championed my no quit attitude. I'd gone on this trip intending to show off how well I could snowboard. They're mostly between 30 and 40 with one or two older guys. I think I'm a pretty good snowboarder for an old man. I was later told that my skills on a board weren't what impressed them. What impressed them was how hard I worked at getting up after falling in the deep snow. How I would never quit or take a break. I fell a lot, and it's very hard to get up from deep snow with your feet strapped to a board. While we were sitting around the hot tub at the end of our first day, I recall one guy, Chip Duffie, commenting, "There is sure no quit in John Kuby".

These guys have no doubt that I have it in me to beat cancer. But then again, none of us really knows what it's going to take. I worry about what I'll be like when the pain comes. My mantra is "no quit in me," but I haven't really been tested yet. We will see. Another thing I worry about is getting totally wrapped up in myself. I already feel that I'm becoming very self-absorbed. Even more self-absorbed than I usually am. Which, on a scale of one to ten, is an eight. Ask my brother and sisters.

Maybe I do need to go inside myself to gather my resources, but it may not endear me to Linda, my family, my staff, or anyone else on my support team. I guess I can trust that they'll be understanding and forgiving. I hope I don't get too lost in myself. Today I told my office manager, who had recently beaten cancer herself, that I was sorry I hadn't been more empathetic when she was fighting cancer. She said that she hadn't noticed because I'd done all that she'd expected of me. As she was recovering, I'd allowed her to work on her own schedule, when or if she wanted to. She seemed appreciative, and it made me feel better about myself. Maybe I have it in me to say and do the right things, even when I'm not feeling as empathetic as I think I should.

Our kids are talking about coming to see me before the operation. They're living all over Canada – in Toronto, Ottawa, and Vancouver. Linda wanted to know if I thought that was a good idea. I think now is a good time as I'll probably be in no mood for visitors after the operation. At that point, all I'll want is undivided love, care, and attention from one person. Linda. Now she wants to know if I'm going to be grumpy like my dad was when he was sick. Or like my son, Mike, when he's in pain. Linda isn't sure she can love a grumpy me, but I'm not worried. She'll fake it if necessary.

HOW DOES IT FEEL?

It hurts a bit, but not too much. Just a constant reminder that the tumor is there. The pain is located about where my throat and tongue constrict to send down the food as I swallow. Just above the Adam's apple from the outside. I feel it on the inside left side, on the wall on the back of my throat. It's a bearable pain, but I can feel it most of the time. When I clear my throat of phlegm and swallow, the pain gets sharper for a moment while the phlegm goes past what feels like an inflamed part of my throat. It's more unnerving than painful. I called the doctor's office about it and they phoned in a prescription for Tylenol 3. I take it, but the pain still seems to be there.

Eating is a bit of a problem. I can eat, but it hurts as I swallow. I have to swallow toward the right side of my throat. Who knew you could do that? There's still a bit of pain with each swallow. Solid food goes down OK. Best if it is soft like pasta or cooked vegetables, which slip down easily. Little bits, like rice, and even parmesan cheese, can get caught in the phlegm somewhere past the raw part of my throat. They become irritants and cause me to clear my throat repeatedly as I eat. Sometimes I need to cough in order to get it clear.

It's a challenge for Linda to figure out what meals to make that I can eat. She's doing a great job. I do eat, and I do enjoy my food, but it's a bit of work to get it down. It also hurts a bit to drink water. It helps to tilt my head to the right as I swallow water. But hey. I'm brave and can still drink my beer like a man.

I drink smoothies in the morning. Yesterday we bought a Vitamix, a $600 blender. Each of our kids owns a Vitamix and uses it all the time. They think it's about time we came around.

Linda is concerned about my losing weight. This is the first winter that I haven't ballooned up to 175 pounds, from the 165 pounds I usually weigh when I'm in shape after mountain biking all summer. Since before Christmas I've been working out with weights, seriously watching my food intake, and I've stayed just over 165 pounds. I've also been doing resistance training and high-intensity workouts three times a week, 20 minutes a day, at home. That, with a lot of stretching ("yoga sorta," I call it). In the winter, I often snowboard for a couple of hours at a time at one of three river valley hills here in Edmonton. I try to do some form of meaningful exercise every day except Friday. We don't know if it's my hard work and discipline or the cancer that's keeping the pounds off. Probably both. I'm not sure if I look like a "fit old man" or a "sick old man." I do know that I'm about 162 pounds and my pot belly is almost gone. I look trim. That's a good thing.

Linda's managing her weight and health too. Along with walking, she's going to Curves three times a week. She also does Weight Watchers and keeps me on the Weight Watchers plan. We're both healthy going into this. Linda looks great. I still have shallow values, so that matters.

We'll know the PET scan results on Monday and hopefully will soon have a biopsy and a treatment schedule.

I haven't been at work since "the news." I'm grateful that my staff is taking care of the business.

We're planning to go to Vancouver for a family visit soon; I have close family and relatives there. We'll fly three of our kids there and enjoy some time together before my operation. My brother's son and his wife have a new baby for us all to meet. Maybe my Mom will come from Winnipeg. It'll get her out of the seniors' home for a while. She's 94 and still quite active. It's all good.

APPRECIATING LINDA

One of the themes percolating through the comments that I received from blog readers was how lucky I am to have Linda supporting me through this. They were right to remind me; I need to be reminded to not take her for granted.

A female friend once asked Linda, "What does it feel like to always be the most beautiful woman in the room?" I doubt that Linda had an answer, other than to say that her twin sister has often been in the room with her. It's not how she thinks of herself.

It's how I think of her. Being shallow and all. I'm always proud to be in a room with her. The most beautiful woman in the room in every way that a woman can be beautiful. What truly makes Linda beautiful is how thoughtful she is, and how smart. She brings something special everywhere she goes and to everything she does. I'm a lucky guy. She's a wonderful companion. I'm thankful that she's in my life. My cancer will be hard on her. It's not fair. She's going to need support buddies too.

Thank you, Linda. You make me a better man. I love you.

STILL WAITING

No news yet. We saw my family doctor yesterday and he had my PET scan on his screen but no radiation oncologist's report on it. So, there was nothing much he could say. We just have to be patient and wait.

Meanwhile, the T-3's are working and the pain has abated so I went back to the PlayWorks office today just to check in. My staff was beavering away, getting it done, and letting me know that it's not necessary for me to be working. Good to know.

I have many feelings about having cancer. My big upside feeling is gratitude. Gratitude for the expressions of sympathy, the shared wisdom, the advice, and the prayers from the many people reading my blog. I've also received many emails and phone calls, a few visits, and some nice hugs. I've been bathed in positive attention. Almost enough to kill the cancer.

OFFERS OF HELP

I've received many offers of help, some of which have been very specific.

My son Mike, the one with the business degree, who's now studying photographic arts in Ottawa, immediately offered to come home to help out with the business if I needed him. Jeff, my son who lives in Vancouver, offered to help me stop drinking by quitting with me. He figures it has to be the drinking that caused the cancer because it's my only unhealthy habit. Maybe we can just cut back together and not really quit. Oh right, we're not halfway guys.

Mike and Jeff, Jeff's girlfriend, Connie, and Linda's kids, Kyle, Kirsten, and Kirsten's husband, JP, all had a big "come together" Skype meeting to hatch a plan for a get-together in Vancouver. My sister in Vancouver, Callie, and her husband, Tom, don't know it yet, but they'll be hosting this get-together in their big house in Belcarra.

A few people offered to get me medicinal cannabis oils. Marijuana may not cure cancer but it might take my mind off it. I'm up for anything that might get me high and cure cancer at the same time. Maybe they are on to something. Or maybe just "on" something. We'll see.

The staff at PlayWorks have all stepped up their game and have said, "John, you take care of you. We'll take care of the business. We've got this." I've barely gone into the office, or done much work, since I found out about the cancer. Everything is going well. Sales are up, and it looks like we'll have a very successful summer. We have lots of good projects on the go. My staff is taking care of everything. I'm grateful. Many of the manufacturers we represent have also stepped up and have said that they'll do what they can to help us through this.

The F'n riders, my group of mountain bike riding buddies, who know me to be constantly in need of help with everything from a flat tire to a broken light on my helmet, immediately assumed I would now need a different kind of help. Many of them have said they are there for Linda and me if we need any work done around the house or yard. Hmmm. I can always think of a few things around here that I don't know how to fix. One of my Pow-Pow Crusher snowboarding friends, Jesse Hahn, offered his truck any time we needed it! Other Pow-Pow Crushers have emailed and called me with offers of help with business issues. Antoine Palmer, a business guy with a lot of connections, has introduced me to someone who will be very helpful for my business.

Ashley Ryniak, one of the Dirt Girl mountain bikers,

offered the gift of music. She's always sending good tunes my way and has promised to seek out some healing music, specifically for me. Another friend promised a new song every day on my blog, but that'd require too much of his time and attention. A new song now and then'll be good enough for me.

Ryan deMilliano, a Pow-Pow Crusher who also does video work, very generously offered to shoot my next snowboarding video, "Grey on a Tray #3." He, Linda and I drove to the ski hill in Jasper to spend a day videotaping me snowboarding. Apart from shooting it, Ryan will also have to edit several hours of footage down to three minutes. I'm proud to say I already have two snowboard videos on YouTube. The one that was shot when I was 64 has 154,000 hits!

A number of friends have focused on my comfort and well-being. Deanne Morrow, a good friend of Linda's, who's a quilting artist, is making me a quilt with bikes on it. I can't wait to see it. One of the Pow-Pow Crushers, who owns Range Road, a fine dining restaurant specializing in locally sourced food, offered a catered meal delivered to our door. Graydon, Linda's ex-husband, and his girlfriend, Nan, did the old-fashioned thing. They made a delicious stew for Linda and me and brought it over to the house.

Brianne Nord Stewart, a young friend of our kids, and Daniel Arnold, my nephew, both of whom work in film and television in Vancouver, each did the same great thing for me without being aware that the other was also doing it. They put me in touch with a mutual friend of theirs who'd survived tongue cancer – Gary Harvey, a TV and movie director. Gary is two years into his tongue cancer experience and is now back working very successfully. We've only exchanged two emails, but I'm certain that knowing him will be helpful for me. I can tell from the emails that tongue cancer is harder than hard. He also conveyed confidence that I'll get through it, but I'll be a changed person. His email to me was full of emotion. He'll be a powerful ally in my getting through this shit.

WISDOM, ADVICE AND PRAYERS

I have been getting a lot of great advice in the comments section of my blog. The best advice and wisdom came from people who'd either had cancer or some other illness that was equally hard to manage. Here are some of the highlights.

Learn to breathe to manage the pain. Take a serious yoga class.

Take one day at time. Know that this too will pass.

Be grateful every day.

Know that my life has changed forever.

Don't second-guess my medical team.

Do everything I can to build up my immune system and to help myself recover.

Cut out sugar.

Keep my weight up. *Boost* and *Ensure* nutritional drinks could be helpful.

Keep up the protein intake.

Do resistance exercises so I don't lose too much muscle.

Meditate.

Trust my virtues.

When dealing with the health care system, ask questions. Don't be afraid to look stupid. Look out for number one.

Journal about my illness.

Know that the "battle" analogy is not accurate. This is more like an endurance race that will feel like it will never end.

Be aware of Linda's needs too.

I especially valued being told that people whom you assumed would be there for you may be just too busy with their own issues to be available at this time of crisis. That saved me a lot of unnecessary disappointment. I appreciated my friend Greg Matthes's honesty when he wrote that he'd be there for me no matter what, "as long as it doesn't involve time, effort or money." That is so like Greg. So like me too. No wonder we've been best friends since we were teenagers. He's never forgotten what a smart-ass I was when we first met.

Many people promised to pray for me. I'm thankful to be included in their prayers. I don't know if there's anyone hearing or answering prayers, but I don't doubt the power of reaching out. However, I don't resonate with the message from fundamentalist Christian friends who've told me that I need to come to Jesus now in case I meet my Maker soon. While I appreciate their caring, I don't believe what they believe. If there is a God, I believe He's a forgiving God, one who would forgive me for not believing in Him. I'm also betting that if there is a heaven, that my living a good life will earn me enough points to get in.

Many friends have reminded me of times I've triumphed over adversity in the past. The Pow-Pow Crushers expressed their admiration for my ability, at age 68, to comfortably hang out with 35-year-old studs for five days on a cat ski and snowboarding trip. My friend, Rocky, called me "Kubinator, the Cancernator."

To keep my head from becoming too big for my hat, a number of people remarked on the irony of me, a constant talker, getting cancer of the tongue. When I mentioned all the complimentary messages I'd been receiving, Lorna's wise husband, George Hornbein, not so subtly reminded me, "What else are people going to say to you, John? You told them you have fucking cancer."

A PROFOUND EXPERIENCE

One day at breakfast in Vancouver, my son, Mike, Linda's daughter, Kirsten, her husband, JP, and Linda's son, Kyle each took turns telling me how they felt about me as a parent/role model and how I had impacted their lives. It was quite moving. There were tears. Many tears. It's a blur to me now, but the emotions were powerful. Kyle shared how I'd been more of a friend to him than a stepfather, and he appreciated that. Kirsten told me that my vibrancy and resilience were an inspiration to her. She also seemed to enjoy my sense of humour. I've always appreciated her laughing at my jokes.

The tears really came when Mike spoke emotionally about how I'd always been his hero, and how I was even more of a hero now. JP, Kirsten's husband, talked about my sense of adventure and referenced a couple of daring bike rides I'd taken him on.

Linda talked about how much faith she had in me to get through this. She's seen me go through many other challenging times in our life together.

From each of them, I understood their fears for me, but also their faith that I'd be able to handle whatever was in store. I could feel their love, respect, and admiration for me. It was powerful to hear what I meant to each of them.

In one important way, this cancer experience has been a real blessing, since one of the deeply embedded concerns in my life has always been my ability to measure up. I never felt that I measured up to my father's expectations of me, and as a kid and as a young man I craved his approval. As a family, we joke about my brother being the favourite son, and I've always been Ok with that. My brother is a very cool guy. But, even now, as essentially an old man, I wish my Dad could see the man I've become. Not that I blame him. I really was irresponsible and self-centred. He hated that in me. I always forgave myself. In my mind, I had time to grow up. These acknowledgments from Linda and especially our kids seemed to demonstrate that I eventually did grow up. Sure, I'm a bit scatter-brained, and I don't know how to fix anything, but I'm actually a high-functioning person. I've done some good stuff with my life. Lots to be proud of.

Am I the only one with doubts like these?

BIOPSY

Things are moving along. They do the biopsy early in the morning on Wednesday. Once I have the biopsy results, my doctor will outline the course of treatment. We've heard nothing about the PET scan results. I could worry if I wanted to. It helps that the Tylenol 3's are working, so there's very little pain.

My staff is taking care of things at work, so as they instructed me, I'm just taking care of myself now. I'm trying to get in as many dinners with friends as I can before I can no longer eat. I'm focusing on the good things. I was bike riding with the F'n Riders last night. Nick Croken took great pictures of me climbing hills.

I recently bought some good books on pain management in preparation for what's to come. My favourite is *Full Catastrophe Living – Using the Wisdom of Your Body and Mind to Face Pain, Stress, and Illness* by Jon Kabat-Zinn. I'm about to take an on-line self-care program for cancer patients through Inspire Health Integrated Cancer Care in Vancouver. I want to be informed and prepared.

I was at the hospital by 5:30 in the morning, put under anesthesia at 7:20, and woke up an hour later. By then, Dr. Harris, the surgeon, had spent 10 to 20 minutes exploring my throat and esophagus.

Before he put me under, I had a chance to tell him that he'd once worked on Kyle, Linda's son, who had a lymph node problem, and that Graydon, Kyle's dad, had asked me to tell him how impressed they'd been with his work and his bedside manner. The doctor was noticeably pleased. Maybe the compliments bought me an extra five minutes of looking around in my neck. Who knows?

I woke up from the anesthesia with pain in my head, face, shoulders, and neck muscles. So that gave me an opportunity to practice my self-massage and breathing techniques to relieve the pain. I think it sort of worked. Thankfully, I'm now on *Tramacet*, the equivalent of T3s without the constipation, and am feeling pretty good. Woozy good.

An unusual upside of the morning's experience was getting to know Oscar, the nurse who looked after me. It started with him complimenting me on being in such good shape, which quickly became a comparison of fitness regimes and the beginning of a new friendship. He's 44 years old and a lifelong soccer player who is now a road bike enthusiast, big time. He is currently looking for a winter sport and was inspired by my learning to snowboard at 50 with our three sons, ages 10 to 13. He has two boys, 10 and 12, who snowboard and ski.

But when he takes them to Rabbit Hill, our local ski hill, he just sits in the chalet and drinks coffee. So I'm now going to teach him to snowboard. He's very excited about it. Me too.

In exchange, he's going to teach me how to speak Spanish. He's pumped to teach me his first language. Linda will be happy to have me learn it as she already speaks Spanish very well. It fits with her plans for travel in our retirement.

Oscar is from Columbia with a fascinating story of how, as a 20-year-old, in order to save his life, he quit the Columbian army and left the country with only a backpack full of possessions. He eventually backpacked around much of the world and met his lovely Venezuelan wife (I've seen photos) in the United States. He had no papers to allow him to stay in the US, so eventually they came to Canada. Canada's gain. The US's loss. Screw Donald Trump.

Oscar is a model citizen and now owns a new house in suburban Edmonton, right near Elizabeth Finch School, where PlayWorks has built a fantastic new playground. And I now have a new friend.

Oh, and yes, I remembered to ask Dr. Harris when we'd know the results of the biopsy. He told me we'd get together in two weeks to discuss it. "That fast! I'm so impressed." He responded with a surprised, "Really? Most patients want the results in three days." Flashing my Kuby smile, I explained, "Yes, me too, but I've been well-prepared by your nurses to expect much less. How much better can we do?" He answered with his Dr. Harris smile, "Two weeks is fast for Alberta."

So there we have it. A bit of "Hurry up and wait." Nonetheless, I feel like I'm being well cared for.

SICK OLD MAN

Last fall I wished I was 155 pounds, my ideal playing weight. (I'm usually 174 pounds this time of year.) I'd been trying really hard, since last fall, to keep from gaining winter weight. In fact, I'd been trying to get below 160 pounds. Congratulations are now in order, thanks to cancer. Be careful what you wish for.

My weight was 165-ish all this winter and then it settled at 162 over the last few weeks. Not bad, I think. I looked like a fit old man. But yesterday it was at 157. And, today it's down again to 156. Linda says I'm looking like a sick old man. She'd been warning me all winter that being too skinny is not a good thing. "What if you need some reserves? Then you'll wish you had that pot belly back." She was right, as usual.

I'd been finding it harder and harder to eat. For a while the T-3's took away the pain associated with swallowing, so eating got a bit easier. It still hurt, but not much. The *Tramacet* I was given after the biopsy seemed to work better than the T3's. I was taking one every five hours. Then, a few days ago, I choked on a couple of pills I was trying to swallow. I had to hack them back up. It was scary.

Even worse, I scraped the side of my throat that was easiest to swallow on. Now it hurts to even swallow water or saliva.

For a few days, I wasn't even drinking beer. Then I found that if I upped the *Tramacet* to two every four hours, it killed most of the pain. I can now eat, drink, and swallow but I have to be careful. Now I'm relying on painkillers. Some of my support buddies were worried about me driving my car while on *Tramacet*, but it doesn't seem to affect me. I assured them that I'd watch to see that it doesn't. I've always been good at driving slightly inebriated. Maybe this is the same thing?

Another good thing about *Tramacet* is that it dulls the aches and pains that I often feel in my shoulders and neck. That is a welcome relief as those pains which have been with me most of my adult life had been intensified by my swallowing problems. I've also been using yoga, relaxation, and meditation techniques to relax those muscles and to take away the tension and pain. I'm pretty sure I am going to need to get really good at some of these techniques.

How am I going to keep my weight up? I've started a new campaign to get back to and stay over 160 pounds. Strange to be trying to gain weight. Breakfast is usually a smoothie made in our new Vitamix with lots of fruit, veggies, and protein supplements. I've found that porridge goes down easily as well. We also add yogurt, berries and hemp hearts to jam in as many good things as possible. Lunch is now a bottle of *Soylent*. Mike turned us on to *Soylent*. It's supposed to be a good meal-replacement drink, better than *Boost* or *Ensure*. The taste and texture are OK and I find that I can use it to help me swallow pills.

Linda is suspicious of food promises so she's doing the internet research on *Soylent*. Maybe she'll find something better. For dinner, she's figured out how to make meals that are high in protein and vegetables that go down well. Taking the *Tramacet* an hour before I eat helps the meal go down without pain. We've been out for dinner with friends recently and I've managed to eat the meals, although with difficulty. It hurts to swallow, but a tasty meal and good company help me overcome the discomfort.

A point of pride. I actually have some muscles under that fat I was carrying. I'm able to do 4.5 chin ups. I started at 1.5 before Christmas. And I can do 45 push-ups. Started at 13 before Christmas. Pretty good for a sick old man. To keep in shape, I also intend to keep doing resistance training three to four times a week, along with some yoga. I'm not sure if biking at the intensity I used to ride is good for me. I find that, even though I might feel strong while I'm riding, a long ride tends to kick the crap out of me. I have trouble recovering the next day. I'm going to have to learn how to ride only as hard as my body can handle.

Generally, I feel more tired than usual. I go to bed a bit earlier and wake up a little later. Guess that happens when your body's fighting cancer.

MEETING GARY

While visiting family in Vancouver, Linda and I and my 30-year-old son, Jeff, were fortunate enough to have dinner with Gary Harvey, a busy guy who gave us two hours of his time to talk about his experience with tongue cancer.

Gary is 53 years old and a TV director who needs his voice to make a living. Gary's surgeon had been able to save him from the worst, losing his tongue, but the whole experience seemed pretty traumatic. He lost 70 pounds, but he's gained 20 back and looks good. Three years after losing 90% of his tongue, he's talking fairly clearly and is working again. Amazing!

He's thankful that his surgeon was able to keep 10% of his tongue and his larynx. Otherwise, he could be feeding himself through a tube. He had a muscle from his leg grafted on to extend his tongue so it works for swallowing and talking. As it is, eating is not easy. The work his tongue would ordinarily do he sometimes has to do with his fingers or fork. Yet, it's his life, his new life, and he handles it with grace and ease. What a classy guy.

With only 10% of his tongue, Gary learned how to talk again. Yes, sometimes it's hard to understand him and I had to ask him to repeat himself occasionally, but in our lively conversation he did most of the talking. He gave us a sense of how cancer will dominate my life for a while, maybe for a long while. We learned a lot about what I may have to deal with, and about some of the concerns I'll have in the long run. For instance, dry mouth is common with throat cancer and it leads to problems with your teeth. Dental care requires more attention now. Taking care of myself day to day just got more complex.

Talking to him also made me feel somewhat hopeful. He told me that this is going to change me. Maybe even for the better. So far, I have to acknowledge some pretty profound things have happened to me since I was diagnosed with cancer – mostly in my relationships with other people. It's not all bad.

My son Jeff sat across from me while I talked to Gary. There were a few cathartic moments when Gary talked directly to me, cancer survivor to new cancer patient. When I looked over at Jeff, he was crying. I was deeply touched by his fears for me and tears of sympathy. I was glad he was there.

Gary's a wonderful example of someone who's handled his tongue cancer gracefully. He's now an important role model for me.

WHAT THE FUCK IS GOING ON?

It's 3:00 in the morning. In eight and a half hours, I will meet with my surgeon to get the results of the biopsy and to talk about a treatment plan.

Lying in bed tonight, wide awake, I experienced a moment of real panic for the first time. For a short while, my mind was filled with a profound fear. Why me? What the fuck is going on? How bad can this get? All accompanied by shortness of breath and a flushed feeling over my body.

This had actually all started with good thoughts. Thoughts of appreciation for my tongue and what a miracle it was. Then, I started to think of myself without my tongue. That was almost unimaginable. Too scary to even think about. I started feeling panic and needed to talk myself down from the fear. This is how I did it.

I let myself sit with the fear for a while. Just let it wash over me without trying to stop it. Then I asked myself. "What's the worst that can happen?" The answer was, "It's never going to be as bad as you fear. You're being cared for by the best doctors. You're resilient. You've been through fear-inspiring/life-changing issues like this before. You'll adapt. This is life. You are you. You have Linda, you have your kids, and you have the rest of your family and friends taking care of you. Your staff is taking care of your business. Your responsibilities are being taken care of. All you have to do is get better."

"Breathe deeply and slowly. Feel the fear, and let it go."

The panic didn't last long, but it made me realize that I'd been floating above my situation and maybe not facing the reality of what was really happening. The fear went away, but the questions remained. What is "better" going to look like? This is going to change me forever. I know that's true, but how? Is it going to be painful? Will I be gripped by fear? Will I be resentful? Am I going to be speech-impaired? How bad? What will it take to recover? Is cancer going to take over my life?

How will it affect my relationships? How do I function without my smile, or without talking? My tongue gets me out of more trouble than it gets me into. Will I still have a smile in my voice? Will I still have a voice?

All fear-inspiring thoughts. All about unknowns. Maybe my doctor's visit today will bring answers? Probably not. This is just something I'm going to have to watch unfold and deal with day to day, one step at a time. If it takes six months, or a year, or more, to rebound from this, then so be it.

How does this compare with the pain and suffering other people go through? I just learned that my brother, who's four years younger than me, is suffering in a whole different way. He has tinnitus, a ringing in his ears that won't go away. Loud noises really bother him. To the point where he couldn't join our family at a restaurant in Vancouver. Yet every day he has to go to work and deal with all the crashing and banging at the loading docks and depots he works at. He drives a truck.

Two of my sisters had ulcerative colitis. I've had it too but not as bad as theirs. They've both lived through way more physical pain and suffering than I ever have. And they're both OK now. One of my staff suffers from migraines. Headaches worse than I've ever experienced. And she still manages to get her work done. I wonder if I could have worked with those headaches?

We all know people who are suffering, or have suffered. It's part of life. I'm not immune to it, I guess. None of us are. But our suffering is our own. This is going to be mine.

WE WERE NOT PREPARED FOR THIS

We met with Dr. Harris, my surgical oncologist at the University of Alberta Hospital yesterday. It turns out the panic I felt the night before was justified. I don't know what we expected. We'd always assumed that this was going to be hard. My family doctor had said that this was an ugly cancer. But still…

Linda and I came out of our meeting feeling like we'd been hit by a truck. Since then, we've been trying to process the information and to get adjusted to our new reality. I took notes and Linda recorded what Dr. Harris said. We went over everything together this morning.

The tumor is large. It covers half to three-quarters of the back of my tongue and the top of my voice box. The cancer is also in the lymph nodes on the left side of my neck. It is an advanced stage cancer: Stage 4. Seventy percent of patients with this type of cancer present themselves to oncologists at Stages 3 or 4 because the tumors are usually hidden deep down the throat where it's hard for family doctors to notice or to find in the early stages.

The good news is that the cancer is not at Stage 4A, meaning it hasn't spread to the lymph nodes. The other good news is that this is a common, treatable type of cancer (squamous cell cancer). It is HPV 16 Positive oropharyngeal cancer, caused by a virus called HPV (Human papillomavirus). Another bit of good news is that I'm a non-smoker, so treatment success improves because of that.

However, the choices for treatment are between hard and hard, with no guarantees of anything.

The first option is surgery – removing the entire tumor from the tongue and lymph nodes. My whole tongue would be removed at the same time. Linda and I sat and listened in a state of shock as the doctor talked about taking my tongue out. It's an extensive surgery involving 18 to 20 hours in the operating room, followed by two weeks in the hospital and four weeks rest at home. Then there'd be a round of radiation treatments for five days a week for six weeks, supported by three to six rounds of chemotherapy. Radiation treatments take 15 minutes per day at the hospital. The chemo and radiation are used to clean up any microscopic disease left behind that might develop into new tumors. The procedure can be started four weeks from now, if that's what we chose.

What the fuck? Why would we choose this? It involves taking out my whole tongue. Really? My whole tongue?

Our other hard option involves intense radiation and chemotherapy. It would necessitate six weeks of heavy doses of radiation to kill the cancer. Treatments would start a month from now, followed by three months to a year of rest and recovery. If the radiation doesn't get all the cancer, I still might require surgery. If surgery is necessary after radiation, it'll be hard to do and fraught with difficulty, due to the scarring left by the radiation.

Linda and I looked at the pros and cons of the two options. In the case of surgery, the advantage is that it's a bulky tumor and surgery works better on bulky tumors. Doctors here are quite familiar with this surgery and are among the best in the world. The University of Alberta hospital does a high volume of this surgery. On the down side, this is very extensive surgery. It involves the complete removal of the tongue, pharynx, and voice box. If we go this route, the tongue would be reconstructed from a muscle taken from the leg. It would extend down to the windpipe, which would be closed off. I'd end up with a laryngectomy, a hole in the windpipe to breathe through. I'd also have a swallowing tube that I would eat through, with difficulty. This is a gravity system only used for liquids and maybe very soft food. I think I would also get a feeding tube through my stomach. I'd have a speaking valve in my throat to create sounds. My speech would be garbled. Remember, no tongue. I'd be able to manipulate the valve with my fingers but it'd be difficult to make intelligible speech.

Gruesome. Better than dying, but jeez.

As for the radiation/chemotherapy option, the advantages are what the doctor called the functional results or quality of life impacts. The tongue, or most of it, would be preserved. My speech would be good, but my eating would probably be compromised. I would eat through my mouth but it would be challenging. Soft foods, eaten slowly. Five percent of patients who go this route still have to use a feeding tube to the stomach two years after the therapy is over. The tube gets put in before radiation because radiation will also make it harder to eat. As said earlier, if the radiation doesn't work, then it'll likely be very hard to go back and take the cancer out with surgery, maybe impossible. But clean-up surgery could work. It worked for Gary. If I do radiation and chemo, then our surgical oncologist would still monitor my progress in case his services are needed. We'll see the radiation and chemo people next week, likely Friday. They do a PET scan about three months after the radiation to see if the cancer is all gone. What if it's not?

Radiation is very hard on patients. The fatigue is challenging. Some people develop radiation fibrosis, which means that the muscles around the swallowing tube freeze up. That could mean using a feeding tube, all the time, for the rest of my life. There are lots of potential short and long-term side effects to do with swallowing. This can result in quality of life issues that the doctor declined to talk about, saying that the Cross Cancer Institute would discuss these with us.

Based on a recent large study, the survival rate is about equal for either treatment – 80%. Survival means five years cancer free. The choice might come down to quality of life issues further down the road.

My case will be presented to a board of three surgeons and four radiation oncologists from different hospitals in Northern Alberta for their review and recommendation. That happens on Monday this week or next. Our doctor thinks they'll recommend radiation/chemotherapy because of the functional outcomes and the equal survival rates. When Linda asked which option he would choose, our doctor, a surgeon, answered that if it were him or his family, he'd probably opt for radiation/chemotherapy, not surgery. We'll have a better sense once we meet with the Cross Cancer Institute. We still have a week or two to make a decision.

Now what? I've processed the fear and anger, emailed my family, slept on it, read the notes again, listened to the tape recording, talked with Linda about it, cried with my son, Mike, and have written a blog about it. I'm about ready to accept that this is my new reality. It's going to be hard. But there is no quit in me. I don't have a choice. Well, not a good one anyway. Either way, I go on.

FRIENDS AND FAMILY
HELPED ME COPE

Feeling sorry for myself is kind of over. Writing about it helped sort things out in my mind. And making it into a blog was much more powerful than simple journaling. I was blown away by the readership and response. Knowing so many people were reading my words validated my writing about my experience and it validated my life and my worth. It was comforting.

Now I feel obligated to overcome this challenge. I'm the main guy in this story; I have to become the hero, the one that overcomes against all odds with the help of my trusted sidekick, Linda.

Friday, after meeting the doctor, we were feeling like shit. But that evening there was a party to attend if we wanted to. Even though I wasn't quite up for it, I decided that I really wanted to see some of the Pow-Pow Crushers who would be there. So we went. It was the 37th birthday party for Pete Wardell, a Pow-Pow Crusher. It was also a celebration of his having run the Boston Marathon last week and of his having come to Canada from New Zealand ten years ago. I'd met Pete and some of his friends some years ago when Linda took a sales training course with them. I got to know him better recently as one of the Pow-Pow Crushers on a Cat Ski Trip. Very cool guy. Someone I'm proud to know. He does business development with a major construction contractor, Chandos Construction, in Edmonton. I'm always flattered when he calls to meet up for lunch or coffee. It was his party but Pete made time for me. He'd been following my blog so he knew some of what I was going through. He took me aside, put his hand firmly on my shoulder, looked me in the eye, and told me sincerely that I was a significant role model for him. He said, "John Kuby is the 68-year-old I hope to become. All the positive things I am doing now in my life now are what will help get me to where you are." This was a well-placed compliment from a consummate salesman, but I chose to believe him. I was touched.

Pete is also an inspiration for me. He ran his Boston Marathon in three hours and two minutes. It was only the second time he had run one. This guy is fit. Also, he's a good snowboarder, a husband, and a proud father. And he had over a hundred, young, hip, cool, successful-looking people at his party. He's miles ahead of where I was at his age. Shortly after the party, Pete emailed and asked if I wanted to get together for coffee, backing up what he'd said about doing whatever he could for me. He's a true Pow-Pow Crusher – a guy who lives close to the edge, committed to success in every aspect of his life. I also talked to other Pow-Pow Crushers at the party, especially Antoine Palmer, the head Pow-Pow Crusher, and his wife Niko. Antoine had just had a preventative operation on his gums that hurt like hell, so we talked about pain. I'm starting to notice how little I think about the pain other people go through.

We left early because I was tired, but I'm glad I went. There were people at the party, whom I barely knew, who were reading my blog. The party was the beginning of getting over the shock from my doctor's visit. The next day a good friend, John Tansowny, called and asked us to dinner with another couple we kind of know, Dwayne Kushniruk and his partner Gay. I felt like shit but we went. Again, I'm glad we did. These two guys are my age and very successful. Guys who have made, lost, and again made way more money than I can even think of. But here we were, the guests of honour. Dwayne, the host, served up a "gourmet, home cooked meal." A meal that was "to die for." I ate heartily despite my throat hurting. The warmth in the room was exactly what I needed.

For entertainment, these two couples were gracious enough to watch the initial version of my new snowboard video, *Grey on a Tray 3*. on a huge TV screen. Dwayne is also a snowboarder, so he was intrigued. We watched it four times and then watched my earlier video a couple of times. Just what I needed. As we left, Dwayne, a big, strong, fit-looking man, took me aside and said, "I want you to know we're there for you John. If you need anything, anything, just call. We're moments away."

And so the mental healing continues.

I slept well for four hours that night, then I got up and did a great yoga session and was able to get back to sleep afterwards. When Linda woke up, we made love for the first time since getting the cancer news. It was fantastic. We lay in bed for a long time and listened to a mixed CD of our favourite love songs, mostly light jazz. Love songs we often enjoy listening to on Sunday mornings. The song, *Fearless Heart*, made Linda cry. The touching refrain of the song, by our favourite singer, Lynn Miles, "I wish I had a fearless heart" made it possible for us both to finally have a cry together. I told her I would have a "fearless heart" so she wouldn't have to. That might not be true, but it sounded good at the time.

I also had great conversations with my kids on the weekend. On Saturday, I called Mike to find out how the year-end showing of his class's photography had gone. It happened Friday night at his photography school in Ottawa. He was pleased with the evening, but not overly. Yes, people liked his work. Two of his photos were chosen to be featured. He probably should have been ecstatic, but he has very high standards for himself. Also, he has no community in Ottawa and he noticed that all the other students had friends and family around them. In Edmonton, he's connected to a big community.

I know he misses that. He's coming home for the summer partly to be here when Linda or I need him. Our talk about his issues and, of course, mine, was good. It was a healing conversation.

My other son Jeff, who lives in Vancouver, had sent me a rabid email late on Saturday night. He'd been reading my blog late at night and had gotten angry and upset because my getting cancer seemed so unfair. In the morning, he realized, as I have discovered, that in the dead of the night things can look pretty bleak. He'd calmed down by the time we talked. We decided that the best thing he could do for me was to just be the best Jeff Kuby and the best damned playground sales person possible. Jeff used to work for me selling playground equipment in Manitoba, but has since moved to Vancouver to sell for a company that represents many of our product lines in British Columbia. When I talked to him, he was working on a big project. He sent me the playground design he had prepared that day. It's really good. Jeff's like a lot of young people I know these days who are struggling to find themselves. Except that Jeff is lucky enough to have a calling – designing and selling playground equipment – and he's being paid to do what he loves.

That afternoon a young friend, a kid like Jeff, 30 years old or so, called to see if I wanted to get together with him for coffee. Jesse Hahn is a Pow-Pow Crusher who keeps in regular touch with me. Not yet as successful as he's going to be. Jesse's still struggling to find his groove in terms of a career, but is still a very cool guy. We went to a movie and then for coffee. Coffee involved stories about some of the crazy adventures of his youth. Jesse reminds me of a young version of me. Except that I was never the kind of guy who took time from his life to be with someone in a life crisis. Yesterday afternoon, he took me to his Bliss Yoga class. It was great. I'm now signed up for Bliss Yoga three days a week.

My mother, who's 94 and very aware, called to say she's been reading my blog, worrying about me, feeling helpless, and doing some crying. She also told me how proud she was of me and, of course, how surprised she is by the number of people reading and commenting on my blog. She said she had trouble imagining me without a tongue. Me too, Mom. Me too. Later she emailed me from her *iPad* and told me that of course my Dad had loved me, even though he treated my brother better, and that he would have been proud of the man I had become. A mother knows what a son needs to hear.

Linda's mother and I talked too. She's sharp, like Linda, and fun to talk to. I think my blog has shown her a side of me she wasn't aware of. She too is surprised by how many people are reading and commenting on my blog.

That gave rise to some reflection and I came to realize that the people reading my blog were all smart, caring, and active people with whom I had at some point connected at a deeper level than just being acquaintances.

For some reason, I'd invited them into my life or vice versa. In fact, I'd actually started inviting people into my life on purpose when I was in my mid to late 50s. I'd always had friends, but for most of my adult life I was such a workaholic that my young kids used to tease me that I only had one friend, Norm. They only knew of Norm by reputation because he'd moved away. I had no time for friends.

Then, when I was 58, my high school had an amazing reunion. I attended with some curiosity about the people I would meet again, 40 years later, and came away in awe of how strongly I felt about my old friends, and how strongly some of them felt about me. So I decided to keep in touch with them. Many of them have commented on my blog. After that, I slowly but steadily reconnected with a few more people from other walks of my life when I was in my 30s and 40s. And I decided to actively create more friends. That is where the F'n Riders and the Pow-Pow Crushers come in.

I've always envied my brother for a lot of things, not the least of them was having a great group of long-time friends in Vancouver. Most seemed to be from a group of hockey friends with whom he'd played since he was in his 20s. That never happened to me. I'd played on a variety of hockey teams until I was 50 or so but never the same team continuously. I always took years off and when I started playing again I just joined another team, like a hired gun. No friendship group.

The F'n Riders is an informal group of mountain bikers I joined when I was 56. At the time there were maybe six or eight people. All good riders committed to a friendly but challenging two-hour ride every Thursday night, followed by beer. Now the group has grown to 25 or so guys, and some women, all committed to the same thing. And we're all much better riders than we were back then. Or maybe it's the bikes that are better. Anyway, we're all glad to be F'n riders.

The Pow-Pow Crushers? I've had the privilege of joining them on what has become an annual five-day cat skiing and snowboarding trip to the back country near Nelson, BC. The guys are between 30 and 40 with a few older guys, but none who are in their sixties. Except me. I'm the odd man out when these guys talk music, TV shows, and movies, but it's a hoot just listening to their macho tales and trash talk. They're great guys, in the mold of my friend, Pete Wardell. Antoine Palmer is the guy who organizes their gatherings along with his friend, Joey Hundert. Those guys are masters at making and keeping friendships. I'm in awe of them.

So it goes. Friends help. There are friends supporting my cancer adventure from many other walks of my life. Relatives, plus the people I know through work. There are also the people whom I know through Linda. Wow, that girl knows a lot of people. She really likes people. I, on the other hand, only like the people I like. I do like a lot of her friends though.

We all make friends as we go along. It's easy to let them slip away. My advice is, don't. Take the time and effort to stay connected. Ken Friesen, a good friend from high school with whom I reconnected at the reunion, is in town today, so he called me. He came over for dinner tonight. Nice.

I'm feeling better about everything. So's Linda. As she pointed out to Ken this evening, "People just adapt. We will too." We are already.

TAKING CONTROL
AND BEING STRONG

It turns out that I'm not seeing the radiation oncologist at the Cross Cancer Institute for another week. Next Friday, May 6. So I know nothing more about my treatment plan or schedule. Looks like I have another month before anything gets done. What do I do for the next month other than worry? Take control and be strong, I guess. And so I've developed a "take control and be strong" program:

1. Gain some weight back. I will lose a lot once I'm in treatment. I was down to 156 pounds. and now I'm up to 160 pounds and climbing. Linda has me on a high fat, high protein diet in the form of a fruit and vegetable morning smoothie, three high- protein meals a day, snacks whenever I can get one down, lots of ice cream and other ordinarily forbidden treats, and five nutritional drinks like *Ensure* or *Boost* daily.

Shopping for high-calorie food and meals has traumatized Linda, a fanatic about healthy eating. She's seeing years of disciplined shopping and eating unraveling before her. It's so counterintuitive. She's worried she'll get fat from just reading the ingredient labels (or, more likely, sampling my meals).

While we already eat very well, we're about to embark on a disciplined program called The Wahls Protocol, a variation of the paleo or hunter-gatherer diet. It's designed specifically for people with autoimmune deficiencies, but it would work for anyone as a healthy healing diet. It's a scientific and well-researched way of using high-nutrient food as medicine. We have the book. We're believers.

2. Get plenty of sleep. I now sleep from 11:30 to 3:30 AM, get up for two hours, do yoga and read, and then go back to sleep for two to three more hours. Sleep is healing, but for some reason, my body doesn't want to sleep more than four hours at a time.

3. Practice yoga, breathing and meditation. I'm about to start my Iyengar Yoga practice at the Family Yoga Centre, not just for the musculoskeletal benefits, but also for the breathing exercises for pain control. I've done "yoga sorta" on and off for years; now I need a more disciplined practice.

4. Get regular Reiki treatments. The one treatment I had from my sister, Shenta, who has promised to provide them regularly, was wonderful. I need to get organized and make this happen more often.

5. Keep up my physical activity, which includes walking (daily with Linda), bike riding (low key for mental

health), and resistance training (low stress but need to keep my strength).

6. Get my affairs in order. Take care of wills, power of attorney, etc. (done). Set up the staff at PlayWorks to manage the business without me (in progress).

7. Refresh my social connections. My blogging community has been a huge source for me. I also intend to stay in touch with my kids, extended family, friends from various phases of my life, F'n Riders, and Pow-Pow Crushers.

8. Plan a Fuck Cancer and Snowboard Video Release Party. Scheduled for Friday, May 27, some of our friends are putting this together for us. Party planning is Linda's least favourite activity, and so she has wisely taken it off her plate.

9. Shrink the cancer with *Phoenix Tears?* OK, maybe this is wishful thinking, but we have friends of friends who have shrunk their tumors with this cannabis product. We have friends helping us with advice and sourcing. What do I have to lose? Err, well — maybe my mind???

10. Focus on projects I want to attend to when I'm strong again. I still want to contribute professionally before I leave this earth and would like to put together some proper research on what kids actually do on playgrounds, and to write a book on effective playground design principles.

NOT A WALK IN THE PARK, BUT MANAGEABLE

Today we had meetings with my radiation oncologist and chemotherapy oncologist as well as other support people at the Cross Cancer Institute. We were there from 10:00 AM until 4:00 PM. Long day. Frankly, the meetings were very reassuring.

The picture our oncology surgeon painted three weeks ago was a lot scarier than the picture we have today. Seems to us that Dr. Harris had focused more on what could go wrong with radiation/chemotherapy rather than the upside, even though that was the option he recommended. He'd given us the impression that the two choices were more equally onerous than we now understand them to be.

Radiation/chemotherapy is not an easy route, but I'm not starting out expecting to lose my tongue. The upside of radiation/chemotherapy, if it all works as expected, is that I could be back to a relatively normal life in less than a year, maybe even six months. How great is that?

The day started with a chance meeting in the hallway with one of the young guys I know from mountain biking, Mike Dickey, who works at the Cross in Radiation. His job is to help the doctors plan and target the radiation treatments. He spent 20 minutes with us and was very reassuring. Molly, a nurse, was even more reassuring. She answered a bunch of our anxious questions, put our minds at ease, and dispelled any doubts we had about going the radiation/chemotherapy route, and about surgery being "off the table."

Dr. Brock Debenham is our radiation oncologist, a cheerful young man, who doesn't seem like a doctor. I found out that his young kids play on the Belgravia Community League playground, which had been designed and built by my company, PlayWorks. It's one of my best playground designs, ever. Good start to our relationship.

All the doctors start out by asking if you know why you are here, and how you got to this point. I think they're checking to see if you've already received the bad news. It seems that I've been more afraid than I need to be. He reaffirmed that the cancer I have responds well to treatment and that the five-year survival rate for patients with my kind of cancer is 80%. For those that don't survive, it's because the cancer has traveled to other parts of the body and cannot be controlled. That's not happening in my case.

Dr. Debenham told us that techniques for handling it have improved, and that it's been regularly and successfully dealt with using radiation and chemo. He assured me that radiation is not painful, that it takes 15 minutes to administer, five days a week, and that I would rest on weekends. The treatment would take six weeks to administer, beginning on May 24 and with the last one on July 6. Thirty treatments in all. He said that there'll be chemotherapy to support it. It would be administered at the beginning, middle, and end of the process. He also told us that I wouldn't feel much for the first three to four weeks, but that the last two weeks would be difficult, as would the two to three weeks thereafter. He said it would take another two months or so after that before I would be fully recovered.

While it's different for everyone, I can expect to feel fatigued and exhausted, especially at the end. Also, the inside of my throat will hurt and my neck and throat will feel like I've had an extremely bad sunburn. There'll also be sores in my mouth, my esophagus will hurt, and it'll be hard to swallow. I may even need a feeding tube for a while, but they try to avoid that if they can. I'll have dry mouth and very thick saliva. Dry mouth could be permanent, depending on how they're able to protect the saliva glands from the radiation. It varies from case to case. Dry mouth can affect dental care and can increase the chances of getting cavities, so we'll be seeing a dental specialist at the U of A. Radiation can also affect the thyroid, which has to be checked twice a year.

Three months after the treatment, they'll do a PET scan to determine if there's any cancer left. He told me there's a 10 to 15% chance that some cancer will be left. That can be dealt with by surgery. The surgery is not a difficult one, in Dr. Debenham's opinion. As he explained, it's a relatively simple neck dissection, as opposed to the surgery originally proposed, a 20-hour process of removing and reconstructing the tongue.

I was relieved to hear that my voice would be OK; the cancer is not on my vocal cords. In the end, I shouldn't have any trouble talking. There'll be some swallowing issues though. My swallowing will be assessed right away and, as treatment progresses, they will measure and track my swallowing abilities. The treatments can also affect hearing so I will need to get a baseline hearing assessment so they can monitor the effects.

The doctor ran a scope through my nose and into my throat to capture an image of the cancer and to project it onto a screen that he, Linda, and I could see. The tumor is a big bulbous protrusion into my throat just above the epiglottis where the food goes down. It was interesting to see the enemy. It's a shiny pink blob. Larger than I'd expected since I can't even feel it in my throat or on my tongue.

We had a meeting with my chemotherapy oncologist, Dr. John Walker, also a very cheerful, charming man, like Dr. Debenham. They make a good team. His kids go to Elizabeth Finch School, where we'd just built a fabulous playground. Good success rate here. We learned that, in my case, radiation is the primary therapy and that chemotherapy is intended to support the radiation. Radiation shrinks and kills the tumor. Chemo improves the cure rate by preventing local failures, spreading, and relapses.

Dr. Walker also affirmed what Dr. Debenham had said earlier about only 10 to 15% of patients requiring salvage surgery, usually for residual cancer cells in the lymph nodes. He's proposing a chemo drug called *Cisplatin*. He has a choice of giving us weekly intravenous low dosages or three high doses at the beginning, middle, and end of radiation. He thinks he will choose the latter. He said that they monitor for kidney issues, which can be a side effect. Another side effect is hearing issues – especially tinnitus, which is ringing in the ears. This is uncommon but it can happen. He says it's reversible. (Tell my brother that. That doesn't seem to be his experience.)

The doctor warned me that *Cisplatin*, which is administered intravenously, will induce nausea. They try to reduce these effects with other drugs administered at the same time. He said he was OK with us to try acupuncture which, according to research, has proven effective. Studies cited by the Canadian Cancer Society show that acupuncture is helpful for easing acute vomiting after chemotherapy. Apparently, regular alcohol drinkers don't experience as much nausea. Which means I'm well-protected! Our brains get used to being poisoned, I guess.

Dr. Walker's suggestion was to stay as active as I can, before and during treatment. Walking, biking, resistance training, and yoga all help with the recovery. Our radiation oncologist also said that there are studies that strongly support exercise during treatment.

Some possible side effects of chemotherapy include damage to the fine nerves in the fingers and feet, which can be reversible if caught soon enough. Immune suppression can also be an issue. I'll have to watch out for fevers and signs of infection. Lots of hand-washing. In addition, I'll have to be hyper vigilant in responding to signs of blood clots, which are rare but still possible.

Dr. Walker had no issue with using a cannabis oil product such as *Phoenix Tears* and thought it might help as a sleep aid, as an appetite stimulant, and for reducing nausea and anxiety.

We left the Cross Cancer Institute tired but optimistic. None of this is a walk in the park, but it seems so much more manageable than the nightmare scenarios presented by the surgeon two weeks ago. It seems wrong that we didn't get the two options presented back to back by their respective advocates. It would have saved us a lot of unnecessary angst.

Oh well. We're both relieved, now that we know my chances of coming out of this relatively whole are very good. In the end, if I do as well as Gary or Freda, an old friend of my mother's, both survivors of throat cancer, I'll be happy. Both of them had complications but are living full lives.

It seems like I get to keep my tongue. Prayers are being answered.

I remember sitting in our surgeon's busy waiting room about two weeks ago, watching a regal looking middle aged cancer patient enter the room with his wife or girl-friend. He was slender, almost frail and weak, yet carried himself in an energetic, broad shouldered manner that commanded attention. He seemed to proudly announce that he was a tongue cancer patient who spoke through a hole in his throat. He spoke to his wife with a garbled sound, seemingly undisturbed by the other people in a waiting room listening.

The T-shirt under his casual sports jacket defiantly read "Fuck Cancer." There he was with his long hair and sports jacket, and a hole in his throat, looking cool and comfortable with who he was, and saying "Fuck Cancer".

That day, as our surgeon talked to us about taking out my tongue, I remember thinking, "I may have to become that guy."

Today I know I won't need to become him, but I think I could do it if I had to.

GETTING SERIOUS

We learned at our chemo education class that the chemo drugs will reduce the white blood cell count, which means a weakened immune system that will leave me vulnerable to infections and illnesses my body would normally be able to combat.

Unknowingly, we'd planned the Fuck Cancer party to fall within the exact days that I would be the most vulnerable to infection – days 7 to 14 after the beginning of treatment. We've decided that the risk of catching something from someone at the party is too high. Also, I'm not quite up to partying. Some days I'm strong and can put in a full day, but most of the time I feel weak and fatigue easily. Then there's my trouble with talking. My throat hurts a bit all the time. I have a sore right where I swallow and it gets worse when I talk a lot. I still do it though. Talk a lot. But the more I talk, the rougher my throat feels and the more painful it gets. It'd be hard for me to be around a lot of people at a party. So the party is off. Too bad. We had a good plan and an impressive guest list going for a while there.

Now our focus is on getting ready for treatment. There's a lot to do. At a recent chemo education class, we learned that chemo works to kill the cancer cells, but it's draining. I may experience some or all of the chemo symptoms, the main one being nausea, which can bother me for a couple of days after the chemo. I have a prescription for a product meant to take care of that. I hope it works. I hate feeling nauseous. I'll also have a lowered platelet count. This means I could experience bruising, nose-bleeds, bleeding gums, and blood in the stool. I could also get numbness or tingling in my hands. Then there could be constipation or diarrhea. And I will probably have sores in my mouth. I will need to rinse every two to four hours with club soda. The bubbles relieve the pain, I guess.

My hemoglobin (the molecule in the red blood cells that carries oxygen) counts will be low, so I'll be tired. The fatigue will get gradually worse over the 30 days of radiation treatment. It'll be at its worst toward the end, especially during the last two weeks, and will continue for two weeks or so after the treatments are over. I'll be fatigued even after the treatment period ends. I could also be short of breath and prone to headaches and/or dizziness.

The good news! The chemo I'm taking, called *Cisplatin* or Platinol, won't make my hair fall out. So that's good. I don't have a nice round head. So, on me, hair is a good thing. That said, I think radiation causes hair loss too so I may still be a bald cancer patient. I sure hope not.

Teeth are also a huge concern for tongue cancer patients. My dentist is a nice lady, but what she had to say about the potential for teeth problems scared me. The saliva glands will not work as effectively as they do now, which means I may not have enough saliva to clean my teeth. They are likely to be subject to more cavities and will decay more easily. Also, radiation causes the bones that support the teeth to lose their ability to heal or grow, which could result in loss of teeth.

My teeth will be vulnerable and it will be up to me to take care of them. Dental check-ups once every three months. Plus, I will have to apply a fluoride treatment every day. It takes five minutes. I have to brush carefully, after every meal, and floss once a day for sure. Never miss. And floss, John, floss. Just another thing for Linda to have to nag me about!

I've been told that my teeth can be saved, and I've also been told that I'll lose them. The truth is probably somewhere in between. No one really seems to know exactly what the radiation and chemo will do.

I'll also experience dry mouth all the time and will have to carry water and other products to counter its effects. Imagine no saliva. I can't imagine. Swallowing is probably hard without saliva.

Next week I get my hearing tested; they want a baseline so they can monitor any hearing loss as the treatments progress. I hope I don't get tinnitus.

In preparation for radiation treatments, I go in on Tuesday to get a mask made up. Moulded to the shape of my face, it's designed to hold my head in place when the radiation is being administered. It directs the radiation to the exact targeted area, the tumor. To aid in this, I'll receive another scan so they can be quite specific about where the radiation is directed. They want the radiation to hit the tumor and miss other critical areas, such as the salivary glands, as much as they can. Reportedly, this is hard to do.

On May 24, I go to an education session on radiation where I will learn about all the risks associated with this treatment. I have now talked to three people who've had tongue cancer. Each of them had problems with their initial treatment. They either had to have surgery after radiation and chemo, or they had to do radiation and chemo after surgery. Let's hope I have better luck. The nurses gave me a list of tongue cancer patients who've had success with this treatment and are willing to talk about their experience. I haven't called them yet. But I intend to.

The radiation/chemotherapy team at the Cross Cancer Institute are optimistic that my treatment will go well. They are among the best in the world at this. They have state of the art equipment and the best treatment drugs. (I wonder if every hospital says that.)

The main goal is to kill the cancer. That'll happen,

I'm sure, but I worry about the damage to me in the process. Everyone warns me about possible complications and side effects. They all seem to be hoping for the best, and at the same time, guarding against, and preparing for, any possible complications. I must say, however, that the team at the Cross Cancer Institute seems reassuringly on top of their game. Everyone is attentive, efficient, and caring. Both Linda and I are amazed at the level of concern, care, and attention we've been getting. I tell people working at the Cross Cancer Institute that if this hospital were on Trip Advisor, they'd get a 5 out of 5 rating from me.

Meanwhile I'm taking care of myself. I'm eating like crazy and my weight is up to 162 pounds. It's hard because I'm not hungry and it often hurts to swallow, but Linda has been making fantastic meals that taste so good that I just eat them. Plus I have a huge nutrient-dense smoothie every morning and drink at least four bottles of *Ensure*-like products a day. That's about 350 calories each.

I'm also going for long walks with Linda every day and doing yoga regularly. Thanks to my sister Callie, who keeps me well supplied, the *Phoenix Tears* is giving me a good seven hours of sleep every night. Every second day, another sister, Shenta, gives me Reiki sessions, which I find to be very relaxing and rejuvenating. They take away some of the constant headaches that seem to emanate from the back and sides of my neck where the lymph nodes are swelling. Linda's cousin, Margaret, a

Reiki master and an energy medicine practitioner, has offered to do a special treatment that she uses to help cancer patients through chemo treatments. Several years ago, I had a serious case of ulcerative colitis, which was miraculously cured by a woman using an energy treatment called "Hands of Light," so I actually believe in energetic healing.

I've also decided to go see Dr. Lin, a Chinese herbalist in Vancouver, recommended to me by my brother whose friend, Rick, recently had tongue cancer. A 40-year-old single father of two boys, he had it six years ago, did not respond well to the initial treatments of chemotherapy and radiation, and was given six months to live. He needed a special, very costly chemo drug from the US and his community raised $65,000 for him. He got the special drug, and he is now cancer-free. However, he's convinced that it was actually Dr. Lin that made all the difference, not the chemo drug. Apparently, when his chemo oncologist saw how quickly the tumor had shrunk, he was amazed.

I now have an appointment. I've heard that Dr. Lin makes up a tea that will help me as I go into treatment. Dr. Lin also wants all of my medical records − blood work, CT scans, biopsy reports, etc. It's interesting that we can get all of those records from the hospital system just by asking. I got them quickly too.

I also have another reason to go to Vancouver. My mom

just flew to Vancouver from Winnipeg with my sister D-Anne to attend our family gathering and to see her first great grandchild.

There's no quit in my mom either.

SEEING THE CHINESE HERBALIST

I'm close to starting radiation and chemo. Chemo starts on May 24 and radiation starts on May 25. Then it's 29 more radiation treatments supported by two more chemo treatments, one in the middle of the process and another at the end.

After a great family visit with 15 of us gathered at my brother's place in Abbotsford and my sister's in Belcarra, I saw Dr. Lin in Coquitlam last Monday evening. He's very polite and deferential, as you might expect of Chinese herbalist, and he's quietly self-assured. He's 60, but looks much younger. He doesn't speak English very clearly, despite having been in Canada for 20 years, but understands it very well. He works out of a spartan office in the basement of his home at the end of a cul-de-sac in a nice neigh-bourhood. His analysis procedure consisted mainly of holding my wrists and reading my aura. I asked if he wanted the medical records from the Cross Cancer Institute. He said, "No." Frankly, I had no sense that he knew how to interpret them, even though he'd requested them. He didn't seem like a medical doctor, but his demeanor and the purposeful way he spoke inspired confidence.

After our session, he showed us his huge supply of herbs and potions and talked about how he had come here from Taiwan 20 years ago. His father had been a farmer. He learned Chinese medicine as a young man after first learning kung fu, and then realizing that he was able to heal with his hands. Dr. Lin's son was at the office helping his dad. At 24, his son is the youngest doctor of Chinese Medicine in Canada.

Dr. Lin let drops of blood out of my thumbs and finger tips and placed a cold, wet herbal compress over my throat, held on with tape, to take away the heat. (I wore it for 24 hours.) He also gave me herbal tea that I was to drink three times a day with meals. Its purpose was to take the heat away and to take the cancer with it. He wanted me to come back next Saturday to see if the tea was working. The session cost me $150.00 and another $440.00 for a month's supply of the tea. A small price to pay for hope.

MY WORLD HAS GONE QUIET

When I arrived home in Edmonton everything seemed OK, but when I woke up the next morning, with the compress on my face, I noticed that my hearing was out of whack. My ears felt the way they sometimes do when the pressure changes as an airplane ascends and descends.

That morning I had a session with an audiologist to have my base line hearing measured. Before the testing, I told the audiologist that my ears felt funny and I wasn't sure the readings she'd be getting would reflect how I usually hear. Sure enough, I failed the tests. After the test, she told me that if I were her patient, she'd be showing me hearing aids. Wow! That was a surprise. I may not have the best hearing but I didn't think I needed hearing aids.

After leaving her office, I put in a busy day at the Cross Cancer Institute getting my radiation mask fitted and doing a scan for the radiation planners to use for creating my treatment plan. By the end of the day, my hearing was worse and continued to be bad for the next few days.

My world has gone quiet. I have trouble hearing Linda

talk even when she's right next to me. I need the TV volume up so loud that it's hard for Linda to watch with me. I can barely hear my stream of pee hitting the toilet bowl or the sound of the toilet flushing. I'm not deaf yet, but I can "hear" it coming.

Why is this happening? None of the doctors could give me an opinion. Was it pressure from the airplane ride? Could be, but the pressure didn't bother me during the flight.

What about pressure from the expanding lymph nodes in my throat? Maybe, but it's affecting both ears equally and you'd think that would cause uneven pressure. Cancer migrating to my ears? Not according to our doctor who has seen the most recent scan. The cancer has not traveled. The herbal tea? Probably not, but when I called Dr. Lin, he said that as a precaution I should stop taking the tea. So I've stopped.

Tomorrow I have an appointment to get my hearing rechecked. I'm sure it'll be worse than the last test. Who saw a hearing loss coming? Nobody. I'm now debating whether or not to go to Dr. Lin for the follow-up visit. My brother, who lives in Vancouver, is now seeing him, hoping for a cure for his tinnitus, which has become almost unbearable. My son, Jeff, is also seeing him for general well-being and higher energy levels. I want to believe in Chinese herbalists, but I'm not sure.

News flash. My family doctor solved the problem. It was

wax in my ears. Yes, wax. The wax is gone now. I can hear again. Why didn't the audiology technician see that I had wax packed into them? But, it's all good now. I can hear again.

As for Doctor Lin, I phoned and told him what was what. He seemed relieved that I didn't blame the tea for the hearing loss. We agreed that I would continue to take the tea for the next week and then come and see him a week from Saturday.

This hearing loss thing has been a stupid diversion. But it's over now. I can hear again and can go back to worrying about my real issues. Like getting ready for chemo and radiation. Sheesh!

LESSONS LEARNED:
OH SHIT, I HAVE CANCER!

- Having even one person you can count on for support can make a huge difference.
- If there is something wrong, tell your doctor.
- If you are in doubt, ask. Don't be afraid to seem dumb.
- Take notes at meetings with your doctors.
- If possible bring someone with you to doctors meetings.
- Treat hospital staff like potential new friends.
- Talk to people who have had the same illness.
- Ask for second opinions and explore options; but involve your doctor.
- Follow your doctor's advice.
- The internet can't see your test results.
- It helps to have a friendship group going into a major illness.
- Eat well, exercise and get plenty of sleep. Help your immune system.
- Attitude isn't everything but it's a lot.

LINDA'S CAREGIVER NOTES:

Uncertainty is hard. The diagnosis of cancer threw us into a quagmire of emotions and a muddle of new jargon. We had to become instant experts on medical terminology, pharmaceuticals, and body parts. It was daunting.

The first hint of cancer sent me to my computer. I felt like a detective trying to figure out what type of cancer John had and what the prognosis might be. Gathering information was comforting to me because it was something I knew how to do.

Unfortunately, the material available on the internet was overwhelming and had to be verified. Incorrect and contradictory information abounded. I attempted to use reliable sources like international cancer organizations, the Mayo Clinic, and the National Cancer Institute.

While we waited to meet the surgeon, I pulled up a disconcerting article that stated a survival rate of 14% for patients with tongue cancer. This turned out to be a prediction associated with men who smoked and drank heavily. Later, I learned that HPV cancers have more positive outcomes. That initial inaccurate information was discouraging.

However, it felt better to be optimistic than pessimistic. I didn't know what was going to happen, but I chose to believe in the best outcome. I chose not to dwell on a negative potential. This is how I try to be – to look on the sunny side of life or to die trying.

I found that people were anxious to help John and me. Most people want to do something to help and to feel they can contribute. I found it hard to know what to ask for, especially for myself.

Scheduling medical visits and procedures, getting to appointments, keeping track of information, preparing food, etc. took so much time. I was grateful to be retired. I can't imagine how I could have done it if I had been working or had young children.

I created a binder for all the documents that began to accumulate – notes from doctors' appointments, prescription information sheets, research papers, and information I found online. My traumatized mind couldn't hold the avalanche of data.

Since my brain couldn't retain information, I would tape record or take notes at our meetings with the doctors. It helped to be able to review the information later when I could process it.

TREATMENT:

I DIDN'T COME
HERE TO LOSE

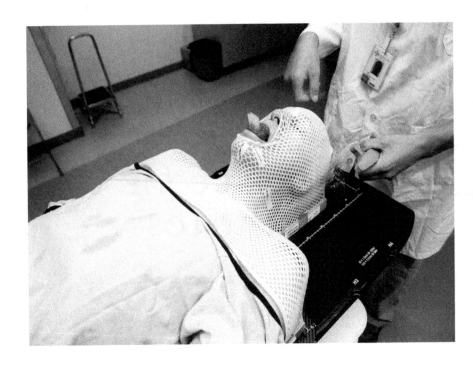

You can view images of radiation treatments (like the one above), chemotherapy administration, nose tube and stomach tube feeding, burning from radiation as well as some recovery photos in the tongue cancer photo essay on:

www.michaelkuby.com | www.noquitinme.ca

CHEMO STARTS TOMORROW.

My first chemo session is at 8:45 tomorrow morning. Four and a half months after feeling my first symptoms and two months after being diagnosed with cancer, I'm about to start treatment. As I said earlier, chemo drugs (*Cisplatin*), intended to support the radiation, are given in three different sessions scheduled three weeks apart. Radiation, the main treatment, is administered every week day for 30 days. The whole treatment plan will take six weeks.

The idea is to nuke the cancer cells and to kill the tumor with radiation. The trick is to inflict as little damage onto the good cells around the tumor as possible. Those who have travelled this road say that both chemo and radiation will be hard on me, each in different ways. The chemo effects can be dramatic but they are short-term; the radiation effects will be more long-term.

I'm going into this knowing that there'll be some damage to recover from. The short-term effects of chemo include fatigue, tiredness and breathlessness resulting from a drop in red blood cells. Nausea and vomiting, which can last for a few hours or a few days, are also common. So is diarrhea or constipation. And I may experience pain in my mouth, gums, and/or throat. Because of a decrease in white blood cells, I need to be very careful not to get an infection; my body won't have the resources to keep it from getting serious. I also need to drink plenty of water to minimize potential kidney damage. And I may need to deal with temporary blurred vision as well as hearing loss, especially in the upper register.

It's going to be hard, but I'll get through it.

To prepare for the chemo, I need to be as healthy as possible going into it. Thanks to Linda, I've been eating a healthy, high nutrient diet. And, thanks to *Phoenix Tears*, I've been sleeping well. Also, I'm pretty fit, with a high base level from mountain biking, snowboarding, and resistance training. To help center me, I've been doing yoga or relaxation exercises every day and going for long walks with Linda in the river valley. I've been well-supported by friends, family, and blog readers, which contributes enormously to my well-being. Plus I've nurtured a positive attitude – I'm going to ride this through to a successful end.

Alternative health care treatments have also helped to prepare me for tomorrow. I've been receiving energy work, specifically to prepare me for the chemo drugs, from Linda's cousin, Margaret, and regular Reiki treatments from my sister, Shenta. Yesterday I had an acupuncture session to boost my immune system. And I've been drinking Dr. Lin's tea, which is meant to take away the heat from my throat.

I have to say that, for the last week or so, I've been feeling stronger than I have since this all started. All the good food, long walks, yoga, meditation, energy work, and generally proactive activity have been good for me. I feel good.

On the day I take the chemo, I have to be well rested, drink plenty of fluids, including ginger ale or ginger tea, ward off nausea with anti-nausea medication and acupressure bands – and have a barf bucket nearby!

Radiation starts the day after tomorrow. I've been told there'll be no symptoms for a while. The first two weeks will be OK, but after three weeks it gets harder, and from what I've heard, the last two weeks will be a different kind of hell. Not going to think about that now. Linda and I are going for a walk. After that, I'll be taking some *Phoenix Tears* – and off to bed.

Am I nervous about my chemo session? Probably, but not that I've noticed. Mostly I'm anxious to get on with it. I'm ready. As Wayne Gretzky said, "The harder you work the luckier you get." I've worked hard to gain some advantage here. And so has Linda. We've earned some luck.

Cancer is Just a Word, Not a Sentence.

In my very first chemo session, I was lucky enough to sit next to a chemo veteran, a sharp young lady named Lisa. She was getting her last chemo for breast cancer. Last of five, I think. She had already had an operation and now has 25 days of radiation to go through. Twice before, while in the chair, she'd experienced bad reactions to the chemo, including vomiting. Today she seemed to do well. Me too.

Sitting there hooked up to our IVs, we compared notes while the technicians first filled me with vitamins, minerals and electrolytes, then the chemo drug, then an anti-nausea concoction. Lisa doodled as we talked, then gave me the page of doodles, and told me to put it on my fridge. Which I've done. The doodles captured some of the things we talked about.

She asked me if I thought I would beat the cancer and I joked that I hadn't come all this way to not win. She immediately looked at me hard and said, "So don't."

Ok, Lisa. I won't.

I've now had one chemo and one radiation treatment. I feel pretty good. Some nausea yesterday and I'm fatigued today but not to the point that I can't function. Got eight hours of sleep last night, so I'm OK.

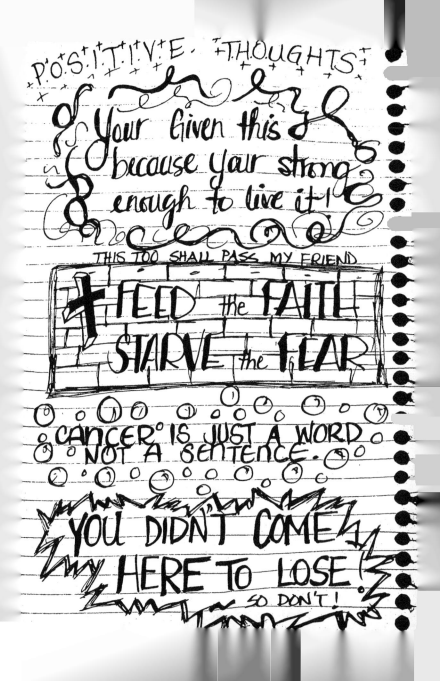

FEELING LIKE CRAP

That was then. Now I'm feeling like crap. I told that to Dr. Debenham, my radiation oncologist today after my fourth radiation treatment, and he said that any symptoms I'm feeling are from the chemo. Radiation issues come much later in the process. (So it's not his fault!) Since the chemo doctor wasn't there to defend himself, I'm blaming the chemo for making me feel fatigued, and often with reflux action going on as well. Acid coming up from my stomach. I threw up last night and then again this morning. Am I feeling sorry for myself? Yes! I'm not feeling pain, but the persistent discomfort is approaching unbearable. I guess the pain will come later when the radiation starts to burn. I wonder how I'll handle that?

The chemo seems to affect everything. Food has no taste. My saliva seems metallic. My body even seems different, almost metallic. I notice it when I take a shower. Even the texture of water and soap on my skin feels wrong. Oh well, this too shall pass. (So I tell myself, but it's hard to believe!)

Wouldn't you know it? What I've been telling myself came true! The discomfort passed. Well, not entirely, but the chemo effect became less pervasive throughout the day and I felt stronger by bedtime. I even went for an hour-long walk last night. Believe it or not, I've become so weak that a walk in nature with Linda has become the highpoint of my days. Not too exciting, but nice.

Now there's a bigger challenge looming. Eating. Yesterday, we met with a dietician who told Linda and me that, at my weight – 160 pounds – I'll need to consume 146 grams of protein a day. Twice what a normal person of that weight needs to consume. As my body tries to repair itself from radiation, it needs more protein. If I can't feed myself enough, then my body will take the protein it needs from my muscles. So, I'll get weaker, and look scrawnier – "not as sexy," says Linda. And it will take me longer to recover. So the goal is to double my protein intake. But the challenge is that my total intake has been dropping because I have no appetite, food has lost its taste, and it's hard for me to swallow. It's becoming very challenging to get food down. Yesterday, it was a bit uncomfortable when I swallowed, but not really painful. Today, it's starting to become painful.

Apart from the pain, the food just doesn't want to go down. Hard to imagine, I know, but it often just sits there at the back of my mouth and the top of my throat. I can push it with water, or a drink like *Ensure*, but even that's hard to do. Even when it feels like I've swallowed the glob of food, it often doesn't actually go down. Jeez! More water. Plus my meals need to be puréed so I can actually swallow them. Last night's meal looked like baby food, but it was protein-rich and almost yummy to eat. But then I threw it all up after trying to swallow too much of it. The same pureed baby food was today's lunch. Not an exciting meal, to put it mildly. Am I going to get through this?

TOO EARLY FOR A WEAK MOMENT

I have to thank one of my blog buddies, Manon Aubry, who is a cancer survivor, for this terse bit of tough love: "It's too early to have a weak moment, John." When can I have one? Never, I guess. No feeling sorry for myself.

I started feeling better yesterday. The chemo-metallic feeling has gone. I'm not as fatigued. I just feel better. Still, the eating issues remain and I guess that will be "the" issue for the duration of my treatment.

I spent the morning at the hospital getting tested for hearing, speech, and swallowing, all of which can be negatively affected by the radiation. My hearing and speech are OK for now, but my swallowing is not. The swallowing issues are caused by the cancer in my throat, not the radiation. Radiation will not have done its damage yet. But the amount of radiation needed to kill the cancer is going to do damage in my throat, and swallowing may become even more of an issue.

They took video x-rays of me drinking and eating from little cups of barium-laced food of various consistencies – from watery to pudding-like. When they showed us video images of my swallowing, you could see the food going down. What they're watching out for is food or liquids going down the airway and into my lungs. Aspiration can happen as the cancer and/or the radiation interferes with the swallow signaling in the throat. Aspirating food or liquid into your lungs is dangerous. It can cause infections that can lead to pneumonia. Not good.

Aspiration's already happening. Watching the x-ray of me swallowing what amounted to a light smoothie, we could see most of the food going down the esophagus, where it needed to go, but there was a little stream of liquid food slipping down the airway toward my lungs. They showed me how to stop the aspiration by doing a short, hard cough at the end of every swallow, to send it back into the esophagus. The best way to avoid aspiration is to avoid thin liquids. Not just beer and wine, but almost everything, including soups and *Ensure* or *Boost* drinks – even ice cream is too watery. They showed us a product called *Thickenup* that we can add to liquids to get the right consistency.

The tests showed that I should eat food that is the consistency of what my swallowing coach calls "nectar" – above watery and below pudding, like apricot or mango juice. It's actually the consistency of my smoothies, so that's OK. Now Linda has to make all of my meals nectar-thick. Go Linda. And I have to swallow properly. Swallow hard to push the initial gulp down, cough to get the part draining into the windpipe up and into the right location, and then swallow again. Each swallow is an action that requires attention. The food doesn't go down naturally. That's why I have to concentrate on doing hard swallows.

I just downed a huge smoothie and a big glass of a watered-up, pureed meat meal from the day before. It wasn't too bad. I'm trying to get up to 3,500 calories a day to keep my weight up. That's a lot for me. Did I get all of my protein requirements from that meal? Not likely. As I've said, I need 146 grams a day. My weight with no clothes on was 154.6 pounds yesterday morning. This morning, it was 153.8. So I lost a pound on a day I thought I'd eaten well. Not good. I've lost 12 pounds since my cancer diagnosis. I'm looking strong but moving toward gaunt.

Last night, Michael, our son the photographer, took a portrait of Linda and me together. We felt we should do this before the "gaunt look" really takes over. The more weight I lose, the worse it gets. The portrait looks great.

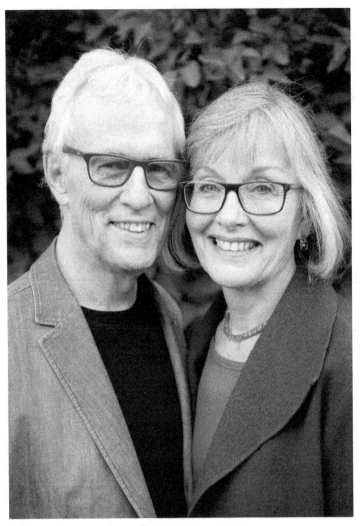

JOHN KUBY AND LINDA RASMUSSEN

Photo by Michael Kuby
From "Tongue Cancer: A Photo Essay"

To view the full photo essay of John's Cancer experience
please visit www.michaelkuby.com or www.noquitinme.ca

Next step in my adventure is a weekend with out-of-town visitors. My son Jeff and his girlfriend Connie will be flying here from Vancouver; my sister D-Anne will be coming from Winnipeg; and Serge Morin, a business associate and a great friend, will be flying in from Montreal. We'd planned the Fuck Cancer party for this weekend and these guys had purchased plane tickets, so why not come anyway? We've also invited some of Jeff and Mike's friends, and of course Shenta, my sister, and her husband Gary, who live near Edmonton.

The intention is to spend Saturday in Riverdale enjoying summer activities. We have six or eight mountain bikes for trail-riding as well as kayaks to take up the North Saskatchewan River and paddle down. And there are endless walking trails. We can also swim in the river. The water is fast but shallow and it's clean enough for swimming. The weather will be nice. Then we'll have a BBQ and an outdoor fire pit for the evening. Gary and Shenta may also perform their folk music for us. It'll be fun.

Now I'm going to make myself a nectar-thick smoothie. More fun!

THE EFFECTS OF RADIATION

The nausea and fatigue from the chemo are gone, but my taste buds seem to have changed, as food is very unappetizing. Even my creamy ice cream is not that appealing.

The effects of radiation are showing up now as well. The biggest issue is dry mouth and sores in my mouth that are somewhat comparable to cold sores. The sides of my cheeks and the roof of my mouth are raw, and the tip and underside of my tongue is sore. I can see small red lesions on the inside of my lips. It's painful but bearable. I can still eat, although it's a chore.

I received prescriptions for a numbing goop to swish in my mouth and a concoction called *Dr. Akabutu's Mouthwash*. I swish it in my mouth four times a day to heal the sores. I've been using it for two days now and I would say it's kind of working but not really. I also have a moisturizing mouthwash that I use regularly to help address the dry mouth resulting from the radiation damaging my saliva glands. I also experience dry mouth symptoms in my throat, which make it hard to swallow. I frequently have thick saliva collecting in my mouth and I have to spit to get rid of it.

The biggest problem is eating. Or not eating and losing weight. As I've said, all the food I eat has to have a nectar-thick consistency. Think a thick milk-shake. I can't drink juices or water as some of it goes down my windpipe and I have to cough it up. Not pleasant. I do drink a very thick mango juice, which goes down pretty easily as long as I tilt my head to the right so it slides down without irritating the cancer on the left side of my throat. I'm guessing that's the cancer anyway; it feels like a raw or open sore.

I don't want to eat. I have no appetite. It hurts to swallow. Not unbearably painful, but it hurts. There's no joy in even eating a bowl of very rich ice cream which would be my favourite thing to eat. But I also don't want to lose muscle or lose weight. I already have. I'm down to 152 pounds and at risk of losing a lot more weight. So I've been cramming in the calories and the protein over the last four days and have held back my weight loss by maybe a pound. That seems like a big accomplishment.

Fortunately, Linda's on top of what goes into my high-protein smoothie, which contains 1700 calories and 136 grams of protein. We put in cottage cheese, Greek yogurt, protein powder, egg whites (raw eggs leave me susceptible to salmonella), flaxseed oil, hemp seeds, avocado, assorted fruits, and greens. It takes me all day to drink it; it's almost like work. In fact, it is work. I keep a glass of water beside me to swish clean my mouth after each gulp. Not having much saliva, my mouth just feels thick with mucus and smoothie that didn't go down. Then I spit into a spit cup and wipe my lips off with a tissue, which goes into a white garbage bag that I keep handy when I eat. Then I get ice cream as a reward – 25 grams of fat per cup and almost 500 calories. Too bad I don't find it rewarding.

For supper, Linda makes pork soup, pulverized and thickened so I can swallow it from a cup like a smoothie. It tastes pretty good. Linda dumps a whack of oil in it to fatten me up. More calories. The dietician at the Cross is impressed with Linda's knowledge of food, and keeps encouraging us. I do my best to get my daily requirements of 3,500 calories, to not lose weight and 146 grams of protein, to not lose muscle. But despite Linda's and my best efforts, I fear I'm losing both.

How do I feel otherwise? I'm OK, but I tire easily, which is frustrating. Sometimes I get irritable. Linda's getting irritable too. She has her own low back and shoulder pain to deal with. Plus, she looks after my diet and appointments, which is almost a full-time job. I'm well cared for and we're doing all right, but we're getting edgy. It doesn't help that I'm absent-minded these days. I recently lost a credit card and a wallet; my forgetfulness has put a bit of a strain on our relationship. Overall, Linda is forgiving, but still...

Now we have another challenge. Linda wears hearing aids and sometimes doesn't pick up on my voice, which has become low and a bit gravelly. It seems that we almost have to be looking at each other in order to communicate. Not a bad thing, but I'm used to just talking and being understood by her as long as she is in the room. So we often get frustrated or irritated at having to make an extra effort to communicate. Also, it's harder for me to speak. It hurts my throat so I don't tend to talk as much as I used to. I notice the pain more when I'm tired, but it's there all the time. So Linda sometimes thinks I'm bummed out because I'm not talking. I'm not bummed out, but I'm definitely not as much fun to be around.

To help with motivation and well-being, I listen to music while I eat. Usually with headphones so I don't bug Linda. She doesn't enjoy listening to music like she used to because of her hearing aids. I'm really enjoying a new CD, called *Weight of the World*, by a band called Western Centuries. It's country music in the old style, beautifully played and sung by masters of their art. The best country album I've heard in a long time. My friend Ashley recently burned a CD for me which she called, "Music to heal the Soul." Lovely songs. Linda does listen to those.

We talked about our relationship last night on our walk in the woods. We've both noticed that we don't talk as much and we don't have as much fun together as we used to. Talking to each other had always been our favourite activity. We miss it.

Other than these relatively minor complaints, my energy level is good and I feel pretty normal.

The next big challenge is my upcoming chemo treatment a week from now.

GOOD NEWS FROM MY CHEMO ONCOLOGIST

We had blood tests at the Cross Cancer Institute yesterday. Then we met with Dr. Walker, my chemo oncologist, and his nurse, Molly. They both think I'm doing well. I was happy to hear that my blood work is normal and the functioning of my liver and kidneys is unchanged from the chemo. Many patients show kidney issues because of dehydration, but I seem to be getting enough liquid. It's probably because of those massive smoothies. Thanks to Linda for pulling together the ingredients and for making me drink them.

I told one of my mountain biking friends that drinking one of those smoothies was like a hard grunt up the switchbacks of a long steep hill. You swallow. It hurts a bit, but not too much. You rest. You know you need to swallow again, so you don't quit like you want to; you go on and take another swallow, and repeat 'til the big mug is empty. This takes up to half an hour. Then you fill up the mug again and repeat with maybe longer rests between mugs. Like I said, it's a grunt. Eating is now an act of discipline. No pleasure. It doesn't feel good, and it doesn't taste good. But it has to be done. It's really my only job right now. I regularly remind myself of mountain biker's rule number five, "Harden the fuck up." Yes, that's right. "Harden the fuck up. You can do this." This is rule number five from a list of 99 rules for bikers. It should be rule number one.

I also have to do swallowing exercises so that my swallowing muscles are strong and work properly. They are kind of like what eating now is for me. No fun. "Harden the fuck up, and do them."

The nurse and doctor both told me I would probably respond to the next chemo the same way as I did the last time. As fatigued and nauseous as I was, they said that my experience was mild compared to what many people experience. Some get sick and throw up a lot. I had acid reflux action, which bothered me a lot, but I didn't get sick. They promised to give me something for the acid reflux this time. They weren't that distressed by my weight loss. I'm now at 152.2 pounds, down from 164 when this all started. They say the weight loss is normal and tried to convince me that it would taper off and I wouldn't lose it so fast any more. That seemed like sugar coating to me. I know full well it will get harder to eat once I've had my next chemo and once my throat starts burning from the radiation.

Today I weigh 151.6 pounds, down a half pound from

yesterday. The doctor says my having been fit going into this has prevented it from being worse. Depending on whether or not I'm tired, I either look fit or gaunt. I can't believe I'm still not down to my playing weight when I was in university. Fifty years ago, when I made the varsity hockey team at the University of Winnipeg, I weighed 133 pounds. I was the lightest guy on the team by 30 pounds. Good thing I was a shifty skater. As it was, I got banged up in the corner by another shifty but much bigger player and was out for the season. I never went back to playing that level of hockey again. Too small.

The next year, I lifted weights and did steroids to bulk up to 148 pounds with lots of muscle. I don't have that much muscle now, but I'm close to the weight I was in my early 20s. By the time I'd hit my late 40s, I'd almost done what most men do as they age – gain a pound a year.

At age 42, when I met Linda, I was a chubby 170 pounds. I've stayed within five pounds of that for 26 years, sometimes up to 175, sometimes down to 165, depending on what regime I'm following. I really hope I can level out to a strong and fit 155 pounds when this is all over.

Ok, now I have to go make my smoothie and start the whole routine again.

More good news! That mouthwash they prescribed – *Dr. Akabutu's* – is working. The sores in my mouth are not as bad now and the numbing goop makes it easier to get the smoothie down past the sores. But I still have to "harden the fuck up" and do it.

Last night we went over to our friends John and Peg Tansowny's house for supper and I couldn't eat the special creamy ice cream they bought for me. What was once a joy has become a discipline, and last night I just didn't have it. Neither the discipline nor the ice cream. Oh well.

I AM NOW RETIRED

I'm very happy to announce that I've just concluded negotiations with a buyer for my company and have now sold my business. I am 68. I am ready to retire. Not having to think about the business while I recover from the effects of cancer, chemo, and radiation will be a blessing.

It's a very big deal – for both me and Linda. We're very pleased to have sold the business to someone who's likely to continue my legacy, treat our staff well, and grow the company. I've known the new owner, Jill White, for over ten years. She owns one of the companies for which we were the Alberta dealer – Waterplay Solutions out of Kelowna BC. They make water spray park components. Jill bought Waterplay ten years ago and grew it from 12 employees to 66. Waterplay is now one of the top spray park equipment manufacturers in the world. She knows our industry and I'm pleased that she is bringing her management skills to PlayWorks and ParkWorks. Good for our staff, our installers, our suppliers, and our customers. And it's great for my peace of mind.

I'm pleased with the deal we struck. Jill was fair and offered us exactly what my business broker told us the company was worth. The negotiations were relatively easy, but the process of validating everything and providing Jill with the information she and her staff needed to do due diligence was challenging and time-consuming. I really need to thank Don Wong, our financial guy, who's been working tirelessly for two months now, including many evenings and weekends, to prepare all the financial records so the transaction could occur. You wouldn't believe how complex the process of valuing, selling and transferring the ownership of a business is. It's a massive undertaking. There are a lot of moving parts and I'm thankful Don was able to take the lead on getting it done. God knows I've been too busy with this cancer thing.

Jill and I had talked about this a few months ago, but when Jill discovered that I had cancer, we agreed to hurry up the process. One of my Pow-Pow Crusher buddies introduced me to John Carvalho, a business broker, who managed the process for us. He was fantastic, as was our lawyer, Ross Swanson. Their insight and attention to detail were impressive. Jill felt the same way about those two guys. Real professionals. Selling a company that you've built over 35 years is challenging. These guys and Jill made it easy. The whole process would have taken much longer if we hadn't known and trusted each other and if we hadn't had such good help.

When they learned about the sale, some of my staff also

stepped up and helped. I think they realized that, at 68 and fighting cancer, I needed to retire. Jill has now met with them and they're impressed with her. She'll be good for the company.

Linda was also a huge help. While she was looking after my cancer-related needs, she was also monitoring all of my business relationships, clarifying everything, giving me advice, keeping me on schedule, and attending every meeting. She was involved every step of the way.

I'm proud to have built a business that is big enough and successful enough to sell. Along with employing 12 full-time staff, we provide business opportunities for a variety of small contractors and their employees who install the products we sell – playgrounds, spray parks, and many other park-related products. Our business coach, Catharine Philips (Wright), told us that only .0048% of businesses that become incorporated ever grow to the size of our business.

It's a major accomplishment to have built a business that's stable enough for another owner to take over, but I didn't do it alone. Key employees have been with the company for ten to 20 years; they built the business with me. Now, my business doesn't depend on me. For the last three months, I haven't been there to run things. My very competent staff ran the business day to day.

Linda and I and our family will do well financially. Jill

is taking over a successful business, and the deal allows us to take our retained earnings out of the business. It's enough for us to live well in retirement on the earnings of our invested capital. We're thankful.

Now I can get on with beating cancer.

MY "NO GOOD VERY BAD DAY"

I guess things have been going too well lately.

Today it took me all day to drink my smoothie. My throat seems more constricted, so swallowing really hurt. Also, my mouth sores are so bad that I just said "Fuck it!" to the instructions on my bottle of viscous numbing goop, which say that I'm only supposed to use it four times a day. I now apply it whenever I want, which is every time I eat something. That seems to work. As long as I don't swallow the numbing goop with my food, I think I should be OK. I just swish it in my mouth to coat the sores and then spit it out. That numbs the sores enough for me to eat.

I ate a lot less yesterday and lost another pound. That pound may have actually been the weight of that huge turd I finally released after having been constipated for the last three days. What a relief! I have never been constipated for that long. Never again. I spent four painful hours trying to release that sucker. I'd been taking *ClearLax* for constipation, but obviously not enough.

The secret, in case you're interested, was sitting on the toilet seat with my feet elevated to the sides on a low stool in front of the toilet. Like the *Squatty Potty*, a new product we saw recently on *Shark Tank*. There will be no next time. Too painful. From now on, *ClearLax* will be a critical ingredient in all of my smoothies.

At my radiation treatment yesterday, they discovered that my radiation mask, fitted tightly to direct the radiation, didn't fit the same as it did at the beginning of my treatments. We had to cancel my treatment so they could make adjustments to the mask. My weight loss has changed my face and body. Mike Dickey, my mountain bike riding friend who works at the Cross Cancer Institute, reprogrammed the radiation. I got the day off but they added on another treatment day at the end of my 30-day program.

I also discovered yesterday that I seem to have sleep apnea. I fell asleep during a relaxing energy work treatment by Margaret Langston, and she noticed that I had moments when I was struggling to breathe. She timed the moments when I wasn't breathing. Up to 20 seconds, then breathing for a minute, and then stopping again. My sister had noticed the same thing when she gave me a Reiki treatment. Gotta look into that, I guess.

Linda was of little help yesterday, when I was in pain, because she was doing her taxes – for the third time, believe it or not. She had entered all of her expense receipts for her businesses (*LegalShield* and the rental unit), and when she saved the *Excel* workbook, all but one of the worksheets disappeared. So she had to redo them. Five extra hours of tedious work. Then when she went to save it, the work disappeared again. Argh!

She'd been working with a program that didn't save the way she'd expected, and so yesterday she found out what she'd been doing wrong and did the work over again for the third time. We allowed her to be grumpy, but that coincided with my grumpiness. Double grumpiness. Things got quite a bit better after she finally sent off the files to her bookkeeper and I finally had my momentous bowel movement. Until the Golden State Warriors lost to the Cleveland Cavaliers. I like the GSW. Oh well, at least we get another basketball game to watch.

On the good side of things, last night I used *Phoenix Tears*, a cannabis product, to get me to sleep last night and I slept very well. Maybe I should be using it more often.

I've been writing this while in my big chemo chair at the Cross Cancer Institute. It takes about four hours for the nurses to administer the drugs intravenously while I just sit here. It doesn't hurt but it's boring. Some people have reactions while in the chair. Not me, at least not this time. My son Michael took pictures of the process, some of which are featured on my website.

ROUND TWO OF CHEMO IS BETTER

I'm doing well, so far. Better than the first round of chemo.

There seemed to be no chemo effect for the first two days, but by the third day, I was getting tired. That evening I could feel my stomach churn from nausea coming on strong – despite having taken three pills in the morning and two at night for the first three days to keep the nausea at bay. I couldn't eat because of it.

This morning, I feel good, but mornings are always best. I managed to sleep through the night without too much trouble. We will see what I am like today. I'm glad to not be experiencing acid reflux. I take a daily pill to prevent it because it was such an issue last time. I also don't have that metallic taste in my mouth or that metallic feeling in my body. I'm thankful for that. Maybe it'll come, but it hasn't so far. I still have chemo brain. Dazed and confused, making silly mistakes. That could also be my normal ADD or just senior moments. But overall, I seem to be doing better than last time. Fewer uncomfortable chemo effects like nausea or weakness.

My swallowing is better than it has been, although I can still only drink smoothies. Thick, no-taste smoothies that are getting boring and challenging to eat. I've been doing swallowing exercises that help get the food down. They also strengthen my swallowing muscles to prepare me for radiation damage of my throat muscles. Evidently, doing these exercises will help with recovery.

My weight seems to be staying at 152 pounds, which is acceptable. I struggle to down all the calories and protein I need. It's fun putting that big-ass smoothie together, but it's a day-long chore to glug it down. It's unimaginable how little interest I have in food. No taste. Slimy texture. Sores in my mouth, difficulty swallowing. No upside except I need the fuel in me.

And now I have a new concern. On the day I did chemo, I got a deep cough in my lungs. Not too bad. I don't cough often. Mostly when lying down and mostly in the early morning. But it's in my lungs. So, we have to be concerned about an infection and possible pneumonia. I was worried and went to the hospital as my doctor and nurses had recommended. They did blood work and a chest x-ray and determined that it was not pneumonia. Thank goodness. So now we monitor it.

It's Saturday morning now. I see Dr. Debenham on Monday. Am I beating the cancer? A few days ago, I needed to have another CT scan to help in recalibrating the radiation. The CT scan didn't tell us anything about the primary tumor, but it did show that the cancerous lymph nodes in my neck are receding. I can also feel that they're almost gone. Dr. Debenham says that that's an indication that the primary tumor is also receding. So there seems to be progress.

I'm on day 17 of 30 days. Thirteen more to go. So far, so good.

More good news. I'm not losing any hair, yet. *Cisplatin*, the chemo drug I'm on, doesn't cause hair loss. The radiation process might result in hair loss toward the end of the treatments. Mostly around the back of my neck where the radiation strikes. Not too noticeable, and it comes back later.

So yes, I guess I'm beating cancer.

TWO GOOD DAYS, AND THEN...

I was super tired and slept most of the day due to nausea. I forced some food down in the morning when I was feeling reasonably good, but after that I slept. I got up and went for a walk with Linda, but I felt weak and we came back early. I moped around for a while, took my anti-nausea pills, and slept again. I threw up a bit before going to bed.

I got up at 9:00 in the evening. It's 10:00 PM now and I'm a bit better. I'd been avoiding eating, but Linda made me a soup. It's there in my cup. Staring me down. I know I have a poor attitude toward my food. I should be more appreciative of the fact that I have food, that I can eat it, and that it will keep me strong. But I'm not appreciative. I'm afraid it'll make me throw up. But I managed to drink the whole cup, three mouthfuls at a time, while we watched a movie.

Sleep last night was fitful. I was awake, off and on, until about 6:00 AM. Dealing with nausea and dry mouth while trying to sleep is frustrating. Dry mouth is what they call too much thick mucus in one's mouth rather than the more fluid saliva that everyone is used to. My mouth is sticky. I have to swish water and spit out the thick mucus frequently to make it feel more normal. At night, my saliva issues get complicated. Sometimes the saliva gets bogged down in my throat and makes me feel like I'm going to choke. I spit into a bucket beside my bed a few times before going to sleep but then later at night I get a different reaction. I seem to have sleep apnea which means that I'm snoring in fits and starts, but I'm also breathing through my mouth, not my nostrils. Sleeping with my mouth wide open means that I wake up with my mouth all dry and parched. To force myself to sleep with my mouth closed, I've developed a technique of lying on my back and twisting a small foam airplane pillow under the back of my head to prop my head up and jam my jaw shut. It sort of works.

At 6:00 AM or so, the nausea got to me and I threw up. Not too much. I was already up at the time, so no mess. Throwing up was a good thing. I went back to bed and managed to sleep through until 8:30 AM.

Now I have to start my day. I feel tired but stronger than yesterday. I still feel some nausea. I'll see how it goes. Chemo effects seem hard to predict.

IT IS WHAT IT IS.

I feel like shit. I couldn't keep food or drink down for two nights and two days this weekend. I just threw up over and over again. I'm dehydrated and I'm losing weight. I was at 152 pounds; I'm now down to 144 and dropping fast. Skinny. Losing muscle.

So...I had to go to the hospital where they gave me fluids via IV today, and will do so again tomorrow. Also, the doctor decided that tomorrow they would give me a feeding tube through my nose to my stomach. So I'll be pumping nutrients directly to my stomach, bypassing my throat. The nose tube will be replaced in ten days with a more permanent feeding tube into my stomach – intended to last for two or three months. While I'm pumping water and nutrients to my body, I will also have to keep eating and swallowing as much as I can so I don't lose the swallowing muscles.

Maybe I'll feel like eating later, but right now I just feel weak and tired. Am I discouraged? Yes. But it is what it is. I need to get my strength back. Maybe the feeding tube is what I need. I sure don't feel like eating now.

After hearing about my chemo issues, Gary Harvey, my friend and tongue cancer mentor,   sent me an email with these supportive and inspiring words: "You're in tough now, John. You've got it though. I was there, exactly where you are. I truly do know what you're going through. Every ugly moment. The hardest fight of your life. You're not alone, my friend. Just a couple weeks left. And yes, at times it feels like you can't make it. And you might even feel like you just want to stop the process and take your chances, but you won't. You can do it. You're in twice the shape I was when I was there. And you're right, it is what it is. It's shitty and it's hard, but you'll get through it. Later I can give you a couple of strategies for the feeding tube. Rest. Don't try to normalize your life right now because it's not normal. And everyone has your back. Unconditionally. Keep your eye on the prize." Thank you, Gary. Great advice just when I needed it.

EVERY HOUR AND EVERY DAY
IS DIFFERENT

On the fourth day after my second round of chemo, I had a meltdown. I was tired, irritable, nauseous, struggling to get anything into me and to have something to vomit up. Dry hurls. I couldn't force myself to eat because every mouthful made me feel like gagging. So, no, I was not drinking those smoothies. To me, they were disgusting. I was losing weight quickly, and for a brief period, I was down well below 140 pounds, looking weak and feeling frail. I was not the hero in this story.

That was a weekend ago – Father's Day. Despite my feeling like crap, we managed to get in a nice long family Skype with the kids.

On the following Monday, the team at the Cross Cancer Institute decided to put me on an intravenous for water. I was getting very dehydrated. I felt much stronger after the hydration, but then I inexplicably had another night of throwing up and dry heaving. My stomach was empty, but I was still retching. I got very little sleep. It wasn't until the afternoon that I found out that the nurses or my doctor had forgotten to administer the anti-nausea medication along with my intravenous drugs. That's why I was dry heaving all night. I was pissed that they'd forgotten and I let the doctor know. He forgave me for being mad and I pretended to forgive him for forgetting. God, I hate the dry heaves.

On Tuesday, Dr. Debenham put a feeding tube through my nose to my stomach and we started my new feeding program. By this time, I hadn't eaten in five days. Being fed through a tube seems to be the only way I can get nourishment. The tube sticking out of my nose might look ridiculous, but it's saving my life. When I started using it, I felt quite frail. Now, six days later, I may look skinny, but I feel quite a bit stronger. I'd been down to 136 pounds; now I'm up to 142.

What I'm feeding myself through the tube is a product called *Resource 2.0* that comes in a 237-ml *Tetra Pak* – like *Ensure* except more concentrated. It contains 477 calories and 20 grams of protein. I just pump it into me through the tube with a syringe. I'm supposed to work up to six tetra-packs of *Resource 2.0* a day. I started at three and now I'm doing five. It takes about half an hour to get one down. I also pump down a syringe full of water before and after each tetra pack, to keep me hydrated. My feeding system consists of a big syringe that I attach to the end of the tube after I've filled it with a *Tetra Pak* of *Resource 2.0* or water. I gradually pump it through the tube in my nose that takes it directly to my stomach. I can't go too fast or I'll feel bloated and it can bring on nausea. Not that alluring maybe, but it's working.

I've set up my big comfy "dad chair" in the living room as my feeding station, where I have my six *Tetra Paks*, a jug of water that I'm supposed to drink each day, a glass, a cup, and my pump and accessories. Then there's the tissues and *Handi Wipes* filling up a perpetually over-flowing garbage can beside my chair. They help me deal with all the phlegm and mucus I bring up continuously, all day long. I'm always horking up big ropes of phlegm and blowing my nose to get rid of mucus. In fact, there are two other garbage can stations in the house – one in the bathroom for when I'm trying to swallow pills, and one by my bed for the middle of the night episodes.

It probably sounds like I'm doing OK. I'm not. I still feel very tired. Linda and I still walk every evening, but the walks have to be short. And I'm always worried about nausea, which means I have to take anti-nausea pills, which is easier said than done. Any time I drink water, it inflames the sores in my mouth, so swallowing pills is hard to do. I use a medicated mouthwash the doctor prescribed to get rid of the sores, but they're still there and they're driving me crazy. Anyway, to deal with them, I first have to apply a numbing gel, which usually brings up a torrent of phlegm and mucus that I have to get rid of. I also have to take a laxative, which means drinking another half glass of water. Unfortunately, the gel doesn't work well enough to kill the pain from water on my sores. It's painful and it's frustrating and I get irritated. Ask Linda.

I actually feel stronger today but for the last few days I've been quite despondent because of how long this whole thing is taking. That's probably a sign that I'm recovering, and now I'm getting impatient rather than feeling grateful. I hope I can get back into a more grateful mode soon. I have much to be thankful for, considering how freaked out I was in the beginning about losing my tongue via surgery. It's all relative. But being human, I seem to be focusing a lot on the negative, despite long periods when things are OK. The mouth pain can be controlled except when I need to take pills or drink my medicine. And the tiredness comes and goes. I now have a pill for when I get nausea. So it's not always bad. I think what frustrates me is that I never know what to expect. Neither does Linda. Every hour and every day is different.

I'm not talking at the moment. Not talking with Linda. Not talking period. It hurts my throat when I talk. I can talk, but I don't; it's too painful and frustrating. Neither of us is used to this, and it's putting a strain on our relationship. A couple of days ago, I actually wrote her a long letter in the middle of the night, all about how I was feeling and what I was thinking. She appreciated it. She told me she already knew how I was feeling and what I was thinking but she was glad I wrote it out for her. I of course already knew that she knew. She knows everything. Still, it was good to write it. And it turns out that both of us had forgotten that the day I wrote the letter was our wedding anniversary, so it was very timely.

So, what's next on the program? They're inserting a feeding tube in my stomach in a few days. Then I won't have this oh-so-attractive nose hose. I'll have a tube coming out of my stomach instead. The operation will only take 20 minutes. So now I'm not talking and not eating. I'm hoping this is the low point but I'm worried that it isn't. We shall see. Just got to conserve my energy and keep going.

I have seven more radiation treatments to go. I'm not sure if the burning gets worse but I think it does. So far, I only have a sunburn-level burn on the outside of my throat, neck, and tops of my shoulders. I put cannabis-infused cream on it and that's soothing. I'm scheduled for one more chemo treatment on July 7, after the radiation is finished. I'm dreading that. For the two previous treatments, I was good for two days, followed by three to five days of nausea and vomiting.

Then we wait to see if the cancer has gone. If it hasn't, then it'll probably mean I'll need some clean-up surgery. I take comfort from the doctors being pleased with what they saw on my most recent CT scan. I can feel the lymph nodes with cancer in my neck have receded – a good sign that the primary cancer has also shrunk.

My next challenge will be learning to swallow again. I can't take the tube out until I can prove I can feed myself.

The doctor expects this will take a month or two. I've lost about 20 pounds. Half of that loss was probably muscle. It's going to be a long road back to riding with the F'n Riders again. But that's my goal.

Well, one of my goals. I have many other goals, like travelling with Linda. We're starting to think about what we can do for travel fun when this is all done. There'll be a time when all this will be in my distant past.

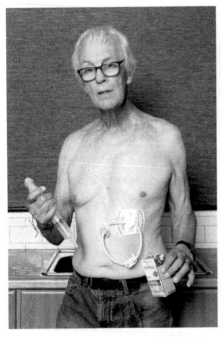
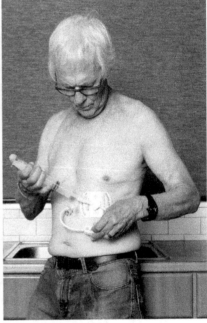

LESSONS LEARNED: I DIDN'T COME HERE TO LOSE

- Use alternative health care, energy work, etc. to keep your immune system charged up to give you strength and aid recovery.
- Allow yourself some weak moments; but get back at it right away.
- This is your "me" time. Do not feel guilty for taking it.
- When it gets bad you really need a caregiver.
- Sometimes it just gets worse before it gets better.
- You might just have to apply mountain biker's rule #5: "Harden the fuck up".

LINDA'S CAREGIVER NOTES:

Getting frustrated is normal. Caregiving is time-consuming, stressful, and elicits "not doing enough." It is a familiar state for many women. One friend told me that the birth of your first child puts women on the path of never-ending guilt.

As John mentioned, we were selling his business at the same time. As he succumbed to the detrimental effects of radiation and chemo, I had to help negotiate the deal, comprehend the massive sales agreement, and keep him on track. I also had to deal with the lease for the building. It was a very positive but also a very anxious time for both of us. Before John signed the contract, it was on me to make sure it accomplished what we had negotiated because John was no longer able to focus on the complexities of the deal.

A major victim of John's cancer was our relationship. His illness shifted the dynamics of how we related to each other. We had weathered many challenges in the 25 years we had been together, but we had always contributed equally to the effort. This time I felt as though I was carrying the burden, despite it being John who had to fight the cancer. I was over-whelmed.

I wasn't always good at helping John find the re-sources he needed, and I was even less effective at reaching out for help for myself. There are a lot of re-sources out there for both the patient and the care-giver. There are doctors, health professionals, cancer organizations, self-help groups, etc. I just had to ask.

It is hard to deal with a grumpy patient. I wanted him to be grateful for what I and others were doing for him. But sometimes he didn't seem to be. I imagined that I would have been a much more positive and optimistic patient but that is probably not true. Still, I wished that John could have been less negative as the treatment went on. It would have made it easier for me! I know what a bitch I am when I am in pain, but it is still hard to deal with another person's bitch-iness.

It is a different experience for each person – the pa-tient and the caregiver. You are going through this together but having very different challenges. This was not the time to work on the relationship, but it was dismaying to feel it slipping away. I missed what we had.

I felt responsible for John following the directions of the health professionals. When he wouldn't or couldn't, I felt discouraged. I remember one weekend, five days after his second chemo treatment, when I repeatedly begged him to drink the smoothie I had made for him. He was shrinking before my eyes and I couldn't get him to eat! I was defeated and scared. It was emotionally devastating to watch my husband fade away. I felt guilty that I couldn't force him to eat and I felt panicky when he stopped eating.

It was a relief when they inserted the feeding tube and I knew that he was getting enough nutrition. Then it was easier for him to take responsibility for feeding himself. I had to tolerate the piles of tissues, the mucus, and the hacking. I felt sorry for him, but I also felt sorry for myself. Remember, I never wanted to look after sick people.

RECOVERY:

LET THE HEALING BEGIN

I CAN SKIP ROUND 3 OF CHEMO

As I've already conveyed in vivid detail, I really struggled with my last chemo session. I'm beyond relieved that the good doctor thinks I'm doing well enough to not need a third one. Thank you, Dr. Walker! There's also a big risk to my doing chemo. My white blood counts are low. They're 1.6, not 4, like we would want. The chemo would likely drive it to down to zero and I would be at risk of a simple infection becoming pneumonia. Death by pneumonia. Not on the "to do" list.

Also, my treatment team said that there's no clear evidence that the third chemo session adds value. Only 60% of patients complete the third round of chemo. In my case, the doctors think "less drama and trauma" to the body is the better choice. If I don't do the chemo then I avoid all nausea and throwing up. Works for me.

The doctors think the treatments have already done their job. The expectation is that, a month from now, when the damage has somewhat healed, they will put a scope down my nose into my throat, and see no cancer. My type of cancer, caused by an HPV virus, is unlikely to spread and, so far as we know, it hasn't spread. That's why they're optimistic.

Three months after my last radiation treatment, they will do a PET scan – to confirm that the cancer has all gone and hasn't spread. This would also involve not finding any cancer in my lymph nodes. The statistics say that there's a less than 10% chance that any amount of primary cancer will remain. There's even less chance in my case since their statistics include a higher-risk type of tongue cancer caused by heavy smoking and drinking. If they find any cancer on the back of my tongue, surgery will be required. There is only an outside chance of that, though, given that my cancer was caused by HPV.

So the radiation and chemo seem to be bringing us to a cancer-free happy ending. Now the healing begins. Now I will need to recover from the cumulative effects of the 30 radiation sessions needed to knock out the primary cancer on my tongue. After the sessions are over, I can expect the burns on my neck to be gone within two weeks and the sores in my mouth and tongue to be gone in two weeks to a month. The feeding tube will remain until I can prove I can swallow and feed myself without it. I need to swallow every day and build capacity; my swallowing coach says the more I keep my swallowing muscles active, the better. I really have to work at it – no choice. This will be my main challenge because swallowing hurts like hell.

The same thing is true for my voice. I can talk but it hurts my throat and my voice has no power. The radiation has damaged my voice box, but it will come back, just like my swallowing will. The mucus build-up in my mouth and throat is expected to go away after a couple of months or so, but I may never be totally the same. Depends on how much damage there's been to my saliva glands. Just as I may always have swallowing issues, I may always have what is called "dry mouth." My taste buds will likely heal more slowly – over the next six months or more.

To help me get through the recovery period, I have my healing team – a dietician, a swallowing coach, the staff at the Cross Cancer Institute, and my beloved Linda. I also have morphine for the pain, and a revolutionary new medication called *Nu-Gel Hydrogel* with alginate for the burns. I'm not going it alone.

I'M GETTING BETTER, SORTA

The burns on the left side of my neck that looked pretty rough a few days ago have healed surprisingly quickly. The burn doesn't look bad and I don't really feel the pain today. It's almost gone. The disgusting globs and long ropes of mucus I keep drawing up out of my throat and into my mouth to be spit out are more predictable and more manageable. Every two hours or so, I spend about ten minutes clearing the guck. Maybe I'm just developing better skills. Still, I thank God for *Handi Wipes*.

My mouth sores are still painful but I've figured out a system for managing the pain. Instead of taking the numbing mouthwash four times day as prescribed, I'm continuing to use it as soon as the numbing wears off. That means eight to ten times a day, and it seems to help. I'm not feeling the nausea that had been part of my everyday experience for a long time. I always had to be aware that I might have to upchuck at any moment. Generally, if I sat up straight and stayed calm it would pass. Yesterday and today, no nausea. A good sign.

Every day I'm able to feed myself five and sometimes six of those *Tetra Paks* of *Resource 2.0* through my feeding tube. My weight is holding steady at 149 pounds. Also, instead of getting up three times in the middle of the night and only sleeping a couple of hours at a time, I slept seven and a half hours last night and only got up once.

I'm noticing some other improvements. I'm able to read about more than sports and the Trump/Hillary soap opera. I actually read most of *The Globe and Mail* yesterday. I also enjoyed watching Milos Raonic's win at Wimbledon, and I'm not even a big tennis fan. Not having read a book in weeks, I almost bought three new books yesterday. One of them was *Dark Money*, a book about the billionaire Koch brothers' manipulation of the Republican Party. I also considered *White Rage* on how African Americans have been systematically held back in the US. Another candidate was *White Trash*, a book about that part of the US population whom the Republicans have been able to exploit against their own better interests. My sense is that the phenomena that these books deal with help explain the rise of Donald Trump. I didn't buy them because I read so slowly that the race issue, for example, might have resolved itself by the time I finish the book! Another modest breakthrough. Linda and I don't normally watch any of the popular TV series, but we've gotten hooked on *Nashville*. We binge-watched two episodes last night. We have to catch up on four seasons! Who knew TV-watching would be a sign of health?

I've also started a modest exercise program. Daily walks or yoga and then adding resistance training with dumbbells as I'm able. The sooner I can ride a bike, the better. Certainly not yet. Yesterday, I actually made a to-do list with about 20 things on it. I haven't crossed many items off it yet, but the point is that, while I often used to make lists, I hadn't made one for over a month.

There are a few things that have yet to change. I can't swallow, am still feeding myself through a tube, and will continue doing so for two to three more months. Swallowing hurts, but I gotta start doing my swallowing exercises. I still have mouth sores, which interfere with everything to do with my mouth, including swallowing. As I've said, they're supposed go away in two weeks to a month. Can't happen soon enough. I still have dry mouth – thick mucus build-ups in my mouth and throat. This could go on for months and months and I may never completely get rid of it. I have a crappy taste in my mouth all the time. Even once I start eating again, which should happen in a couple of months, food might not taste right for quite a while.

I find that I'm easily frustrated and discouraged by how long this recovery phase is likely to take. Then again, I'm generally thankful that I'm recovering and that my cancer experience hasn't been worse. If my doctors are guessing correctly, the cancer is all gone. I hope they're right. We won't know for sure 'til that scheduled PET scan, three months from now.

I SPOKE TOO SOON

It is like I've been lying to you. Right after writing about how things were getting better, I started feeling worse.

The pain has not let up. My first big issue has been managing the pain from the sores on my tongue. My second big issue has been managing the accumulation of phlegm in my mouth and throat, which has been worse for the last few days. I take liquid morphine for the pain, along with that numbing concoction called *Dr. Akabutu's Mouthwash*. No matter how much, or how often I take it, the numbing is very short lived. Maybe half an hour to an hour. *Dr. Akabutu's Mouthwash* is very thick, almost as thick as those mucus ropes I keep bringing up. I swish it in my mouth, coat my tongue, and then swallow it using the swallowing techniques I've been taught. I hate the feeling of it in my mouth but I trust that it's working. Fighting the mucus build-up in my mouth is a constant. Any liquid I use to swish the mucus out and clean my mouth just aggravates the sores. Even water.

This is what I do all day. Fight pain and mucus. That

and managing my feeding and medication program. I nap a lot too. Twice a day sometimes. I'm tired. I'm aware that I'm not doing any of the swallowing exercises that the speech therapist wants me to do. I feel guilty and wonder how much that will impact my long-term recovery. This has all been going on for three or four days and it makes me quite despondent. The good news, if you can call it that, is that I am so tired that despondent seems like normal, so I really don't get too discouraged. Maybe lethargic is a better word than despondent?

Linda has figured out how to organize her day around my feeding, medication. and nap schedule. She talks on the phone a lot to her mom and sister, Lorna. Her mom is always entertaining to talk to and she also enjoys talking with Lorna, whom she's supporting with her heart health challenge. Linda and I don't talk much now. I know she misses our usual chatter. I do too. It is what it is. I can't talk and I have no energy for it. All of my talking is by pen and paper. Today she went on a long nature walk an hour out of town with her friend, Deanne, from Camrose. She's looking after her own needs as well as mine.

Today we were at the Cross Cancer Institute where we learned that my experience of the last few days was normal and to be expected. Many patients have it much worse in the first week or two following the final radiation session, and they get quite discouraged. It seems that I'm on track. I'm faring better than most at this stage.

This stage? They call it the recovery stage. It could continue for another week or two or much longer. It doesn't feel much like recovery. I wouldn't have considered the thick, excessive phlegm that's been plaguing me to be a sign of healing. It's caused by the sloughing off of cells injured by radiation. The radiation attacks fast-growing cells like cancer and, since the mucous cells in the mouth are also fast-growing cells, it kills them off as well. Hence, more gunk in my mouth. The pain and globs of phlegm don't seem as bad today. I hope this isn't just wishful thinking. We will see.

I don't have the energy to do very much. Mostly I just sit around. I am not even going outdoors, despite the weather being nice. So, all I do for fun is listen to music, do some reading, and watch a bit of TV. Getting into *Nashville* has been good for me. It helps the time pass. Pretty boring. Rumour has it that it's going to go like this for a while.

Linda's kids, Kirsten and Kyle, are flying here from Toronto for a week. They're coming to see me, but will also be visiting their dad, Graydon McCrea. They're also driving down to Lethbridge with Linda to see Grandma Scott, Linda's mom, for a few days. I'll be on my own, but it will be OK. My son Mike, who lives in our basement suite, will be around if I need him. Linda needs the break.

MOSTLY I AM TIRED

Not much to report. This would have been easy to write if I weren't so tired. I'm sleeping a lot. Seven hours a night and two, two-hour naps during the day. When I'm not sleeping, I'm not doing much. I haven't been outside for two days now. Mostly I'm managing the usual tedious stuff to do with meals, mucus, pain, and mouth care. When I'm not doing that, I'm reading the book, *Dark Money* by Jane Mayer, which I finally broke down and bought. It's a truly shocking revelation of how the ultra-conservative rich have conspired to systematically manipulate the American political system strictly for their benefit. It's not pretty. Maybe Donald Trump will blow it all up. There are much worse people than him pulling the strings. I shouldn't be reading this now. It's truly unnerving. Maybe it's bringing my energy down.

How am I feeling? Mostly I'm tired, listless, and vaguely out of sorts. I should add the words, "weak" and "vulnerable." I'm moving very slowly. I have to remind myself that this is a stage. I should be glad it's not worse. The sores in my mouth have changed. They're still there, but they're not quite as open or painful. I'm thankful! I hope they'll continue to get better. The mucus in my throat has changed. The gobs and ropes of it that I bring up to clear my throat are much more firm and solid. Maybe that's a good sign? I don't know. It's much easier to manage now. I'm always clearing my throat, which often feels raw and sensitive. Anna, my swallowing coach, has warned me that learning to swallow again is going to be challenging, and this is giving me a glimpse into what I'll be up against.

I am also aware that I'm not doing a great job of managing my teeth. It's hard to brush properly even with my new electric toothbrush. Now that the sores have abated, I should be able to do a better job. I need to remind myself that one of the long-term consequences of my radiation is dental problems. I need to get myself onto a preventative program. As for the burns on my neck, no real issue any more. They looked really bad for a while, but the healing has been surprisingly quick. My weight hasn't changed. I still weigh 149 pounds. I still drink five tetra packs of *Resource 2.0* a day. My only source of food.

Linda's in Lethbridge visiting her mom with Kyle and Kirsten. They get back on Sunday. I hope I'm up for having company by then. Time for a nap.

A WEIRD SCARY INCIDENT

I've just been sitting here feeling sluggish and tired, still dealing with the usual things. Every day seems basically the same. Maybe I'm getting better but I can't tell. Not much to report – until last night.

When I was trying to fall asleep I found that the thick mucus and phlegm that builds up in my mouth was sliding into my throat, causing me to gag. Each gag made me sit up in bed and start hacking and coughing until a bunch of thick mucus was released and I could spit it out. The coughing and hacking hurt my throat. Sometimes it made me actually throw up, which I hate. I would get it under control for a while, start to fall asleep and then it would happen again. I couldn't stop the mucus build-up, couldn't stop the gagging, couldn't sleep, couldn't help but feel panic.

How was I supposed to sleep and spit out phlegm at the same time? Not possible. I very badly needed to sleep, but when I slept I would wake up gagging. It was scaring me. What the hell was happening? This went on until about 1:30 in the morning, when I got up and wandered around, feeling sorry for myself. Linda was fast asleep and there was no point in waking her. Kyle, who was visiting, was up too, so I explained my problem to him. I was feeling trapped, frustrated, and afraid it was never going to end. Nice to have someone to talk to at least.

I decided to try sleeping sitting up in a chair, but that didn't work. I couldn't sleep. Then I tried kneeling forward with my forehead on the couch and my bum on a low stool so I could position a spit bucket below my face. This allowed me to easily spit out the mucus when the build-up was too much. It kind of worked; it stopped the gagging. But I couldn't exactly sleep sitting like that. That's what I was doing at 2:30 AM when Kyle went to bed, feeling powerless to help me. I stayed like that for a while, got it under control and started feeling less frustrated and afraid. Kneeling with my head down on the couch was not exactly comfortable. After a bit of on-and-off sleep, I decided to try going back to bed. So that I could put the spit bucket under my mouth, I lay down with my forehead on a small table near the bed and used a hard memory foam pillow to support my shoulder and to bridge the gap between them. A weird way to sleep, but it worked. I actually slept. Whenever the saliva/mucus build-up got to be too much, I woke up, spit it out, and went back to sleep. Soon it was four o'clock, and I had slept quite a bit. Eventually I got a reasonable night's sleep.

How does this night from hell fit into my progress towards healing? Not sure. I think it's just an incident. A weird, scary incident.

There's some good news. My mouth sores are going away. I'm not generally in pain. I've quit taking liquid morphine as I think that was what was making me so groggy and tired. My big issue is mucus management. Plus my throat hurts when I swallow. It feels hard and raw.

Mentally, I've been feeling kind of out of it for the last few days. Spaced out. I'm hoping that now that I'm not taking the liquid morphine, I'll feel sharper. Socially, I'm feeling isolated. Can't talk with Linda and the kids except with a pad of paper, which is limiting. Not much communication with the staff at work anymore. It's no longer my business. So I'm losing a lot of the social stimulation that I've depended on. All I'm doing now is watching the Republican Convention on TV, and that's not good for anyone's health.

I don't know what I expected to be feeling right now, but it wasn't this.

JEEZ I HATE THROWING UP!

The day went well. More visiting with Kyle and Kirsten. We spent the evening at their dad's. Graydon's an excellent cook. His tradition is that when the kids are in town, he invites us all over for a great meal. Nan, Graydon's girlfriend, Kyle and Kirsten, my son, Mike, and Linda all spent the evening drinking wine and indulging in some excellent food. The food looked so good I felt envious, which hasn't happened to me for a while. I've had no interest in food. Of course, I didn't drink wine either.

It was still a lot of fun and I was able to stay in the conversation with my pad of paper and pen. Toward the end of the evening, I felt some nausea coming on and Mike had to drive me home early.

Within half an hour of arriving home, I had thrown up three times and had completely emptied my stomach. It was unpleasant and unnerving. I have no idea what brought it on; I've been taking anti-nausea pills. Geez, I hate throwing up, especially when there's not much in my stomach to throw up.

I went to bed after that, feeling very nervous about throwing up again and about the problems I had the previous night. I still had stomach churn and nausea, and so, while I worried all night about throwing up again, thankfully it never happened. And the problem I experienced the night before – excess mucus in my mouth slipping down my throat and causing me to gag – didn't happen either. I was very careful not to sleep on my back. Fortunately, there wasn't as much mucus build-up. It seems that, since yesterday, the flow of mucus has decreased significantly. What a relief.

FINALLY, A GOOD NIGHT'S SLEEP

After the last couple of rough nights, I was nervous when I went to bed. It turns out I had no reason to be. I fell asleep easily, and had a full night's sleep. No issues. No mucus build-up, no choking or hacking, and no throwing up. I got up twice in the night to pee, but that was it. Seven hours of good sleep.

The mucus is thickening up, and there's not as much of it. This morning. I can feel the mucus in my throat but I'm not constantly having to clear it and spit out like I did yesterday. My throat's still a bit sore and feels hard and rough when I swallow. We'll be seeing the nurses at the Cross Cancer Clinic today and they're going to want me to start doing swallowing exercises, drinking small amounts of liquid, and trying to speak. I'm ready for this appointment. This morning I did some exercises, drank a bit of chocolate milk, and spoke a few words.

Also, the sores in my mouth are going away, which means I can now use the fluoride treatments for my teeth. I've been neglecting my teeth and from now on I have to be diligent in caring for them. I can't let myself forget that the radiation treatments have made my teeth vulnerable to tooth decay for the rest of my life.

I feel like I've turned a corner. Maybe now I can concentrate on long-term recovery rather than just responding to day-to-day frustrations.

IT SEEMS LIKE THE PRAYERS
ARE WORKING

I'm grateful to the people who've been praying for me. I've had four or five pretty good days in a row. Even better, I've been getting a good night's sleep. In fact, I've been feeling so good that I decided to get on my mountain bike and hit some trails. Yesterday my friend Antoine took me on a ride. We took the tight single-track route across the river from our house that I usually take new riders on. We were on the trail below Ewok Forest and above the river from Dawson Bridge toward the Cloverdale Bridge, and then back along the river. Easy stuff. I'm glad I went. It was fun to be on my bike again.

But, although we were only out for 40 minutes, it was way harder than I thought it would be. I was out of breath right from the start and had to stop frequently to catch my breath and recover my strength. I have a "fall guy" reputation to uphold among the guys I ride with and did have one interesting fall. Don't tell Linda about this one. I clipped my pedal on a stump and went head over handlebars and almost slid off the trail and into the river a few feet away. No damage, but Antoine must have thought I fell hard because he kept asking if I was OK. Yes I was, but the fall did unnerve me. It let me know how vulnerable I am. The main lesson learned is that I have long way to go to get back into the shape I was in before the cancer. I used to be able to ride relatively hard for two and a half hours. Not anymore. I'm a long way from that. Still, I was pleased with my ride and proud of myself.

So, I'm feeling better every day, but I'm still weak. Even during a normal day, I feel a lack of energy and strength. I'll get stronger gradually, but to do that I need to eat. I'm still consuming five *Tetra Paks* of *Resource 2.0*, which is like *Ensure* only more intense. I take them through the feeding tube to my stomach. This gives me 100 grams of protein a day and 2,500 calories. Enough to maintain my weight at 150 pounds but not enough to increase it. What I need is muscle. Which means exercise. But, if I exercise I'm going to have to increase my food intake. That means learning to eat again. The good news is that yesterday I started drinking water again. Not much. Only about eight gulps, but it's a baby step toward eating solid foods. It'll take a month or two to get there. Even if I could eat or drink real food, I wouldn't be able to taste it properly. My taste buds are wonky and everything tastes "off." The "buds" will come back over time. No one can tell me when for sure, but it seems like it could be months.

As for my other issue – mucus build-up in my mouth – that seems like it'll be with me for quite a while. Months, I'm told. I'm always managing the build-up of phlegm and am never without a tissue to spit the mucus into. There are five big boxes stationed strategically around the house, along with three garbage cans that we need to empty daily. I probably use a tissue every ten minutes. Maybe more often than that. Tedious or what? The good news is that I'm not dredging up those big gobs, or ropes, of phlegm like I was before. It used to happen 20 times a day or so, but now it's only a few times. So I'm getting better.

Oh, one other good thing to report is that I'm starting to be able to talk. I get a few words out now and then. Talking irritates the sores under my tongue, but they're gradually going away. The mucus in my mouth also gets in the way, but since that's diminishing, I'm starting to speak occasionally. Linda's happy about that.

I'm still tired most of the time and I nap for one and a half to two hours every day. I'm not what you'd call energetic. Most of my day is spent sitting, reading on my *iPhone* or e-books, listening to music, and watching TV. I look forward to evening walks with Linda, although they usually tire me out.

Over and above recovery, there's still work to do regarding the sale of the business and transitioning to the new owner. And we have a retirement plan to execute.

Also, as I said, Linda's kids, Kirsten and Kyle, were here for a few days for a nice visit. We're actually fairly busy.

Maybe prayers do work.

OUR KAYAKING MISADVENTURE

Noting that I was feeling better, Linda said we should get out on the kayaks like we did last summer. So yesterday morning, when it was sunny and hot, we went. We loaded the kayaks on the SUV and headed off to Emily Murphy Park to put them into the North Saskatchewan River, an hour and a half upstream from where we live. We live just off the river.

By the time we had the kayaks in the water, the sun had gone, it was cloudy, and there was thunder and lightning in the distance. But we checked the weather forecast again and confirmed that it was supposed to be sunny all day with no rain. OK, let's go!

Seeing the rain clouds way off in the distance, we put on our light raincoats to be safe. Good thing we did.

It was nice out on the river. A great way to spend the afternoon. Since my arms were tired almost immediately, I told Linda this would have to be a gentle float downstream even if it took us an extra hour. It started to rain. Not hard, just intermittent. Nice big, soft, warm drops. We pulled the hoods of our raincoats up. By the time we got to the Blue LRT bridge, it was seriously coming down. Oh well. We had our raincoats.

Then, as we approached the High Level Bridge, the rain turned into a deluge. Those light raincoats were not keeping us dry. We were getting soaked. There was also lightning and thunder. We stayed close to the shore so the lightning would hit the trees, not us. A big wind came up making it hard to paddle. Then hail. Quarter-inch hailstones started to land on the covers of our kayaks. We were hoping this wasn't one of those times that the hailstones got as big as golf balls!

Torrents of rain, hail, and wind. The wind surprised us. We were along the shore and I was way ahead of Linda. When I looked back toward the High Level Bridge, I could see that she had pulled her kayak onto a gravel beach. It seemed like she was just going to wait it out. She'd taken off her life jacket and had it strapped over her head to protect herself from the hail. So I turned my kayak back. To my complete surprise, I didn't have to paddle to get upstream to where she was. The wind just blew me along. Against the current; it was that strong. And the rain was not letting up. We sat there on the shore wondering what to do, both completely drenched.

I suggested we just leave the kayaks and hike up to civilization at the top of the bridge. The river runs through a valley in the middle of our city. "No," she said. "This will pass." I didn't argue. Linda is usually right.

Nonetheless, we were scared and in a hurry to get to safety. Home was a long way away and we were going to have to paddle, not float. I was worried about how tired I was going to get. Off we went down the river, paddling hard. The heavy rain wouldn't let up. We were seeing frequent bolts of lightning and for the next three-quarters of an hour we could hear constant thunder nearby. Luckily, we didn't get hit by lightning. The worst that happened was we got soaked.

At one point, I realized that I was actually feeling invigorated, not tired. This beat sitting in my big chair in the living room watching TV or surfing the net. We were on a real adventure. The rest of the trip was just a long, wet paddle. As we passed the James McDonald Bridge and the Low Level Bridge, it was raining hard and didn't let up 'til we got to the Cloverdale footbridge. We were almost home. Fifteen more minutes of pleasant paddling and floating and we were under the Dawson Bridge and landing at the dock near our house.

We'd paddled hard for an hour and a half. I was tired, but I seemed to be getting my strength back. I could see that Linda was happy. Me too. We were both proud of how we'd weathered the storm.

I CAN TALK AGAIN!

I had a *FaceTime* conversation with my mom yesterday. Yes! I can talk again! It was great to be able to speak with her. She was happy to see me and to talk to me – it had been a while.

It's also great to have the energy to engage with regular life. Linda and I had a two-hour meeting with Jill, the lady who bought my business. I enjoyed talking about the business again.

Our evening walks are also getting longer and we're walking at the same pace as we did before I got cancer. The walks tire me out, but we recuperate by watching our nightly two episodes of *Nashville*. While watching an episode of *Nashville* I'll typically use at least 15 tissues. There's always mucus collecting in my throat and my mouth is always full of gunk that I am spitting into a tissue. So that's a constant frustration. What's also frustrating is that if I clear too much of the mucus away, my throat feels raw and I start to gag. Then it hurts 'til more phlegm lines the spot that was hurting. It's a delicate balance. Throat clearing, yes, but not too much.

It is irritating to live with but I try to remind myself that, "this too will pass." I'm lucky that this seems to be the worst of my problems right now. Fortunately, the phlegm problem is not as bad during the day. It's more of an issue in the evening. Maybe the walking triggers it. I don't care. I am not giving up my walks with Linda. Walks with Linda are always therapeutic. Back when we were raising teenagers and managing our careers, our nightly walks were our refuge. One of us would talk about their issues all the way to the turn-around point and the other would get to talk all the way back. It was good. It still is, even though we don't have as much drama to talk through.

I'm sleeping well. Seven hours a night. I wake up once or twice a night choking on phlegm caught in my throat; I've learned to just sit up and clear it quickly. I used to panic but I can cope with it now. And it's happening less and less. I also nap for an hour and a half every day. I seem to need the rest, although I didn't yesterday. Maybe I'm getting stronger.

My weight was up to 151 pounds yesterday. I'm still pumping down five of those *Tetra Paks* of *Resource 2.0* through my feeding tube very day. It takes me about 20 minutes per pack. That plus a fair amount of water before and after. If I do it too fast, my stomach churns and I have to worry about reflux, which is unsettling to my stomach and to my frame of mind.

I'm starting to be interested in regular food though. I'm noticing Linda eating tasty-looking fruits and vegetables and I can smell the really great meals she cooks for herself. Yesterday I saw her grab a handful of almonds and I wanted some.

If I want to indulge this desire, I have to get on with my swallowing program. I'm not working hard enough at it. I'm supposed to be drinking a half cup of water a day and I'm only doing a quarter of a cup. It's hard to swallow. It doesn't hurt too much; it just doesn't feel normal. If I don't manage the swallow properly, then some of the fluid goes down the windpipe and I cough and choke. It can take me 20 minutes to drink a quarter of a cup of water.

My healing team expects that I'll work up from water to juices with a nectar thickness, then on to puddings, smoothies, and eventually soft solid foods. It will be a while before I get to eat real meals, never mind grab a handful of almonds. To reach that point, it could take two or three months or even longer. I should be able to suck it up and push myself to progress faster. It would help if my ability to taste were to come back. Right now, even water has a weird taste.

Until I can eat again, I won't be able to add weight and get stronger. I need to be stronger in order to get back to mountain biking and snowboarding. I'll need more protein if I'm going to exercise hard and build up the muscle I've lost. So my motivation to eat again should be high and it would be if swallowing weren't so uncomfortable.

Is the cancer gone? We don't know and won't know until they do a PET scan in a couple of months. It's possible that some of the lymph nodes will still have cancer cells which will have to be taken out with minor surgery, but probably not. On Tuesday we see Dr. Debenham, our radiation oncologist. He'll be putting a scope down my nostril and into my throat to see if the primary tumor has disappeared. We think it has.

In the meantime, I continue to hang out in my big chair reading, listening to *iTunes*, watching TED talks and podcasts and following the Trump parade. The Edmonton Folk Festival is this weekend. We go every year and have tickets for all four days. We'll see how much of the festival I'm strong enough to take in. Linda's sister, Lorna, and her husband, George, are arriving here today from Atlanta. We're looking forward to their visit and to taking in the festival with them.

Life is good.

DR. DEBENHAM DOESN'T SEE THE TUMOR

Dr. Debenham put the scope down my nose and into my throat yesterday and saw no evidence of the tumor. He admitted that he couldn't see everything, but he felt confident that it was gone. He also felt around my neck for evidence of the cancer that had been in my lymph nodes, but could find nothing.

At this point, there's good reason to believe I'm cancer-free, but we won't know for sure until they do the PET scan in two months. They wait until three months after radiation is over because in the past, up to 10 years ago, they would often get false readings from scans done too soon that sometimes resulted in patients having operations they didn't actually need.

Looking through the scope, Dr. Debenham could see the damage to my throat, which he projected onto a screen. Linda and Mike looked at it with me. The epiglottis, the flap that stops food from going down the windpipe, is damaged and swollen, which is why I have trouble swallowing. It'll take time to heal. There are also sores on my esophagus, and on the other side of my epiglottis, that are like the sores under my tongue. Those sores are going away and should be all gone in a couple of weeks, so I presume those others will be gone too.

Although the damage is extensive, Dr. Debenham was surprised that it wasn't worse. He said that I'm doing as well or better than would be expected at this stage in my treatment. We talked about the mucus build-up. He affirmed that it's from the radiation damage to my saliva glands, which prevents them from producing saliva normally. While I do get saliva, I also get a much thicker mucus which builds up in my throat and mouth. That'll work itself out but it could take a long time. Like up to a year. Hurray. Not.

It was great visiting with Lorna and George during the folk festival. We attended all four evenings and two full days, which was a bit tiring, but I managed. It was also challenging for Lorna, who has a heart problem for which she will soon be having an operation. We were both semi-invalids and Linda and George had to do the heavy lifting. We made sure that we didn't have to do too much walking around the festival site. The festival was fun and we caught a lot of great music, although I was disappointed that there weren't many of my favourite acts. The best act was Passenger. One guy with a guitar, some great songs, and a carefully programed act that had all 13,000 people of the festival hill eating out of the palm of his hand. His music and his rapport with the audience were magic. I had most of his songs on my *iTunes* already, but I was still totally blown away by the live act.

While I didn't like not being able to participate in the eating and drinking, I was inspired to get back to enjoying those pleasures. It's partially up to me to determine how long that'll take. While I'm drinking more water every day to get myself swallowing properly, I need to get my head around eating again. Linda and I have set a goal to be free of the feeding tube by the end of October – in time for us to start travelling and for me to get ready for snowboarding.

Kirsten, Linda's daughter, who's an artist of some note, designed a "countdown" wall chart for me to help us keep track of appointments and other commitments for my treatments. Beside "last day of radiation" on the chart, she wrote that there would still be two hard weeks to get through after the radiation – two more weeks that would "suck and would turn into days where I wouldn't really remember how much any of this has sucked." She was right. I'm in that after period and I can't really remember how much things have sucked.

STILL A LONG WAY TO GO

As positive as things have sounded lately, I'm far from being over this yet. We recently spent time with my dietician and swallowing coach, who made it clear that, even if I'm declared cancer-free, it's still a long haul to recover from the radiation damage. The dietician attributes my feeling strong to being well-nourished by the *Resource 2.0* that I pump through my feeding tube, which enters my stomach a few inches above my belly button and below my rib cage. We now have to wean me off the feeding tube, which they won't remove until I've been eating normally, through my mouth, for a month. Eating normally won't happen unless I work at it. There's radiation damage to my throat that causes me to aspirate when I swallow. When I drink, water goes down my windpipe. This can be overcome with practice and training; eventually I'll be able to swallow without it happening.

Or maybe not. I might always be vulnerable to aspiration. We don't know, and it could take a while to figure it out. Pneumonia resulting from food particles and bacteria getting into my lungs and causing infections is a very real consequence of aspiration.

MORE TO WORRY ABOUT

A key member of my healing team is my swallowing coach, Anna, who has a way of hooking me up electronically so she can monitor the progression of each swallow on a screen that shows the water that enters the throat and passes through. It shows the aspiration when it happens. Recently she said that she's impressed with my progress.

I've been practicing drinking water in small sips and swallowing it in a way that doesn't cause me to aspirate. When I cough during or at the end of a swallow, I know I'm aspirating. I'm already doing it less and less. When I started drinking again, I could only drink a half cup of water a day and I coughed with every swallow, which meant that water was constantly going down my windpipe. It took a week to get up to one cup a day and recently I've gone up to two cups. Now I only cough about every fourth swallow.

The next step toward eating normally is drinking thicker liquids. I've tried mango juice, which goes down well but leaves my throat feeling raw. Maybe it's because it is acidic. I'll try other fruit juices and then soups. I need to keep pushing myself. Before I can eat solid foods, I need to work from thicker fluids such as smoothies toward soft foods. I've tried canned peaches, and they went down OK. I also tried a piece of strawberry. It went down after lots of chewing but I had the same problem as the mango juice – too acidic. The good news is that I can taste the juice and fruit that I've tried. Maybe my ability to taste will come back faster than predicted.

The lack of saliva and the abundance of mucus continue to be a frustration. I spit gunk into a tissue every five or ten minutes. I do less spitting in the morning but it gets worse in the evening. Also, I spit more after a walk or any exercise. It's getting better though. The mucus is not as thick as it was and I can sleep through the night without choking. This is progress.

However, I am still very weak. I get tired easily and usually nap in the afternoon for an hour and a half. I did five push-ups yesterday and maxed out. I used to be able to do over 40. That indicates a huge loss of overall strength and stamina. To build myself up, I've been walking with Linda every day and am starting to go on slow bike rides. Harry, one of my F'n Rider friends, recently took me on a long, slow road bike ride on some country roads. It exhausted me but it was nice to be out riding in the country. Yesterday, Linda and I rode our bikes at a leisurely pace for an hour and a half. That wiped me out, but I have to push myself a bit every day to get my stamina back.

The tiredness I feel differs from normal tiredness. I experience an uncomfortably weird sensation of warm tingly exhaustion in my head and throughout my body. The nurses call it "radiation fatigue." I'm assuming it'll go away as I get stronger. I'm still dealing with learning to eat, mucus management, fatigue – and then there are my teeth. My teeth will always be more vulnerable to cavities because of the radiation so I've been given a strict brushing, flossing and fluoride regime to follow every day. I've not been as disciplined as I need to be, but I'm working at it and I'll get there. Step, step, step. One foot in front of the other.

TRYING TO MAKE SENSE OF CANCER

Cancer is a big topic, having cancer is a huge thing, and everyone's cancer is different.

If you have cancer, it helps to have a family member who takes an active role in helping you get through it. I'd hate to think of what it would have been like for me to go through this shit without Linda and my cancer buddies.

I didn't expect to get cancer. I've only recently learned that over 40% of North Americans get cancer, so my chances of getting it have always been good. However, I used to think I was too healthy for cancer to get to me. I did all the right things – regular exercise, proper diet, good sleep, strong social connections, and I didn't smoke. So I wasn't worried about cancer. Then, when I found out I had cancer, I expected to beat it. I've since learned that beating cancer depends on a lot of factors, many of which are beyond the cancer patient's control. There are many types of cancer and many different causes.

My head and neck cancer, caused by a Human Papilloma

Virus (or HPV), responds well to treatment and has a high success ratio for being cured using radiation and chemotherapy. Lucky me. Most of us have HPV viruses in us. They are sexually transmitted. If you are of a certain age and played around in your 20s, you've got it. Some HPV viruses affect the body's mucous membranes. Genital warts are a common symptom in both men and women. Infection from HPV is widespread. Most often, the body can clear the infection on its own, but if it doesn't, the infection becomes a cancer. Of the 120 strains of HPV viruses, only nine of them cause cancer. My cancer was caused by a high-risk virus, HPV 16. Almost everyone has cancer-causing HPV viruses, but not everyone gets cancer from them. No one knows why.

There are now vaccines that can prevent infection of HPV types 16 and 18. To be effective, the vaccines should be administered before age 11 or 12. Girls generally get cervical cancer from HPV whereas boys get head and neck cancers. Before my getting cancer, I knew nothing about this issue. I'm now an advocate for vaccinating boys as well as girls to protect against HPV's horrible consequences.

I've always been very concerned about smoking as it's a main cause of cancer. Now that I've had cancer I'm even more adamant that my smoker friends quit the evil habit. It can be done. I quit when I was 30 years old after smoking a pack and a half a day for ten years. One of the hardest things I've ever done.

When I found out I had cancer, my instincts were to learn everything I could about it and to find out what I had to do to beat it. That turned out to be a tall order. There's so much written about cancer, it's almost impossible to make sense of it all. Much of what's circulating on the internet is critical of the standard medical practices of surgery, radiation, and chemotherapy. Of course, there's criticism – they're invasive and they have very mixed results. Everywhere we looked – in books, magazines, and the internet articles that well-meaning friends and relatives sent us – there was controversy about typical cancer treatments and the suggestion that there were alternative therapies that might work. The more we read and the more we thought about it, the more we became convinced that alternative therapies were a crap shoot. We were much better off trusting our medical community. My cancer was stage 4, the last stage. Typical of most throat cancers, mine was caught late because throat cancer is so hard for a doctor to see and the symptoms are not predictable. Also, it was a big cancer, 5.5 centimeters in diameter – bigger than a golf ball – and it was growing fast. There was no time for the alternative therapies that were supposed to boost my immune system to fight the cancer, if that's even possible.

It's easy to see why we all hope that alternative therapies will work. Alternative therapies suggest that the body can be helped to defeat the cancer. This thought is comforting since surgery is so invasive and both chemotherapy and radiation are very harsh treatment procedures. But how does one know what alternative therapies to try or to trust? There's no way to know.

If I really wanted to know a lot about cancer, I would have read the definitive book on the subject – *The Emperor of All Maladies: A Biography of Cancer*, written by an oncologist and researcher, Siddhartha Mukherjee, who won the 2011 Pulitzer Prize for this work. I haven't read it because I don't want to know everything about cancer and I don't want to read a comprehensive history of cancer treatments. I haven't been in the right headspace to do so. My brother-in-law, Gary Arnold, is reading it and appears to be fascinated.

We heard the author speak in Edmonton at an event sponsored by the Cross Cancer Institute. The basic message of Mukherjee's talk was that cancer is complex; it changes and adapts and is therefore unpredictable. It affects everyone differently, so it's very hard to predict how it will affect any one individual. That makes it hard for the medical community to create one-size-fits-all treatments and to know what the results will be.

The emerging trend in cancer treatment is viral therapy or immunotherapy, which involves using viruses to trigger the immune system to attack the cancer. There are clinics outside of the US and Canada that offer treatment plans using immunotherapy or viral techniques to beat certain cancers. These new therapies seem to be working for some patients and some cancers and are showing a lot of promise.

Maybe if my diagnosis had been terminal 1 would have explored them myself. The Cross Cancer Institute, where my cancer has been treated, is one of the places that is experimenting with it. My chemo doctor is using immunotherapy with some patients already, but he says it will be a few years before they have a virus to combat my particular type of tongue cancer.

Anyway, as far as alternative therapies go, we decided very early to just trust our doctors and not to second-guess them. If the Cross Cancer Institute, one of the most revered places in the world for cancer treatment, recommends radiation and chemotherapy for me, then that was what I was going for.

We did avail ourselves of Best Doctors, an organization set up to give second opinions. The service was offered by my employment benefit plan. We got all of my medical records from the Cross Cancer Institute (surprisingly easy to get – we just had to ask) and sent them to Best Doctors. They took about three weeks to evaluate them and ended up concurring with the Cross doctors' diagnosis and treatment plan.

Linda and I did feel that it would be helpful to do whatever we could to boost my immune system. People talk about my fighting cancer, but what I've been fighting is not the cancer itself but the effects of radiation and chemotherapy. It's the doctors who've been fighting the cancer.

I'M MAKING PROGRESS

I've been doing my best to progress with eating and drinking without the feeding tube. Eating amounts to being able to slip three or four slices of canned peaches down my throat after chewing them, and drinking amounts to sipping a half cup of water in about 10 minutes for a total of two cups a day. At today's meeting at the clinic, the dietician and radiation oncologist seemed to be impressed with my progress, even if I'm not. It seems that I'm eating and drinking as much, or more, than most patients at this stage. It's now five weeks since my final radiation treatment. I still get all of my nutrition from *Resource 2* through my feeding tube. I've extended my goal for no longer using the feeding tube to the end of November, three months out from my final radiation treatment. That means I have only two more months to train myself to eat and drink all of my calories by mouth.

I can now take two or three gulps or swallows at a time. That is significant progress. I just started drinking small sips two weeks ago. I've also tried eating foods like banana slices, pears, and other fruits, but they get caught in my throat and have to be washed down with water. They also make my throat sore, perhaps because they're acidic. The only fruits that work for me are canned peaches. I'd never thought of fruits as being acidic. Today, I was able to eat a bowl of Campbell's chicken noodle soup. My next step is to try cream soups. The inside of my throat is still quite sunburned from the radiation, just as my neck was. The outside heals quickly but the inside, comprised of much more sensitive mucous membranes, doesn't heal as fast. There's a lot of inflammation.

My healing team think it helps that I was fit going into this, and that I've been active during my recovery. The activity and movement help fight the inflammation, which may explain why I get much more phlegm after a walk or kayaking. The phlegm is a by-product of the healing in my throat. Presumably a good thing. I also get a lot more phlegm after I eat or drink. The team says that this is a sign that I am furthering the healing process by actively swallowing. We left the meeting today feeling good about my progress.

I still tire easily, and I'm often tired during the day. However, I've noticed during my walks with Linda that I'm feeling a more normal kind of tired as opposed to radiation tired. Radiation tired drapes itself over my head and upper body and drags me down. It's a warm, heavy, oppressive feeling – hard to explain since it's not something I've ever felt before. Anyway, the radiation tired seems to be receding. Feeling a normal tired is another sign of progress.

I have good reason to feel optimistic.

HELPING MY BODY HEAL

I was physically fit when I started into this cancer adventure and it has served me well. My radiation oncologist has told us that the reason I'm recovering quickly is my daily exercise and active lifestyle. Being in shape is always a good thing. You never know when you might get sick and need to be strong. I found *Younger Next Year* by Chris Crowley and Henry S. Lodge to be the best book on fitness and health I'd ever read, and I've read a lot of them. It's science mixed with practical advice that's possible to follow if you're committed to fitness. It's also easy to read and inspirational. The original edition was subtitled, "A Guide to Living like 50 Until You're 80 and Beyond," but they changed it to capture a younger readership: "Live Strong, Fit, and Sexy – Until You're 80 and Beyond." There's a men's and a women's version of this excellent resource. I know many people, fit and not fit, young and old, including Linda's 20-something daughter, who've been inspired to turn their lives around by this book.

During my treatments, I kept trying to do some type of physical exercise every day – walking, biking, yoga, and resistance exercise – until the effects of chemo and radiation became too debilitating. The effects of chemo, and later the radiation, made it impossible to exercise or even do yoga for a long time. I didn't have the energy and had trouble concentrating.

As I've said, when I started to feel better, Linda and I began walking together again and we've continued to go out almost every day. At first it was just a slow 20 minutes, but we now walk a brisk 45 minutes. We've also gone out kayaking a few times. Plus I've started doing yoga again. Yoga is great. It helps in so many ways. I do it at home, following a book called *Power Yoga* by Beryl Bender Birch and applying what I've learned at flow yoga classes.

From the beginning of my cancer treatments, I've been using deep breathing, muscle relaxation exercises, and mindfulness meditation to help me stay calm when I'm in pain or in a panic mindset, especially at night. I've often used them to get myself to sleep. I'm thankful that I learned these techniques when I was younger, to help me deal with the chronic muscle tension in my neck and shoulders that has plagued me all of my adult life. I've found that my favourite pain management book is also my favourite book on mindfulness – *Full Catastrophe Living* by Jon Kabat-Zinn. I'm a believer. I've never done much meditation, but I'm starting to now.

What about diet? I've always eaten well. Balanced meals with lots of fruit and veggies. Linda has kept me on track by only stocking the fridge with "real" food. When I first learned I had cancer, we considered two diets that seemed to be immune system boosting – the ketogenic diet and The Wahls Protocol, both of which are variations on the paleo diet. We read the books, and were inspired, but didn't attempt the full-on diets recommended. Life got in the way.

Our dietician at the Cross Cancer Institute told us to just concentrate on getting lots of calories and protein because the radiation and chemo would drain me, and I would need to bulk up and be as strong as possible. So, Linda fed me high fat and high-protein meals and every day I made myself a huge, nutritious smoothie. Turns out I really needed all that fat, protein, and other nutrients.

Cancer consumes a lot of energy and so does radiation and chemo recovery. Even with all of that eating I was losing weight. I started at a fit 164 pounds, with very little extra fat. Gradually I went down to about 150, and then a third of the way through the treatments, when I couldn't eat because of the effects of the chemo, my weight dropped to 141 pounds. For a few days, I even weighed in at 136. That's when I started to feed myself through a feeding tube. Since then, I've been surviving on *Tetra Pak* meal replacements full of calories, protein, and other nutrients. My weight is up to 152 pounds but I won't get any heavier until I can eat real food again

And what about supplements? I was taking *Turmeric*

Golden Honey and *5 Mushroom Blend*. I have no idea if they helped. There's no way to know. I was also taking Korean red ginseng, which I know from previous experience is an immune system booster that does work. It's also an effective testosterone and sexual energy booster, if anyone's in need of that. And what guy isn't?

What about cannabis? We now know that cannabis has healing qualities and is a pain reliever. There are those who even think it can cure cancer, but the evidence is strictly anecdotal. Besides, the dosages recommended are so high that for me it would be impossible. Back when I was young and cool, getting stoned always put me at risk of experiencing serious and debilitating paranoia, the feeling of being left out and left behind. "Cocktail party psychosis," as my brother calls it. I have no desire to revisit that part of my life. But I used cannabis to get to sleep at night and it worked well. I also used cannabis tinctures and cannabis-infused creams as pain killers. I got them from my sister who has joined the ranks of entrepreneurs who are making cannabis-derived products for the new "marijuana is legal" economy. They seemed to work, but when I was in serious pain I relied on the liquid morphine that the doctor prescribed for me.

All of these things seem to have helped me recover from the radiation and chemo. There's damage to my throat that I have to overcome before I can eat again, but I'm confident that I'll get back to normal. Well, not exactly normal. I'm always going to have eating issues. I'll always be managing the effects of radiation on my throat, but the blessing is that I am alive to do it and the effects shouldn't be unmanageable.

There's also a lot to be said for the power of journaling, which is known to be therapeutic. The experience of turning my journal into a blog and sharing my cancer experience with a community of friends seemed to have magnified the therapeutic. It turned my "me time" into "we time." It gave me something meaningful to do during the times when I was feeling shitty. I also have a sense that it kept me from feeling sorry for myself.

I've been inspired by a blog comment from a high school friend, Richard Stecenko, who had cancer several years ago. He said that his cancer progression went from; "Oh shit, I have cancer" to, "Oh good, I'm recovering from cancer," then eventually to celebrating that, "Hey, I'm a cancer survivor," and finally to remembering years later that, "Oh yah, I used to have cancer." I feel optimistic about getting to the last stage.

I AM EATING AGAIN

I am so proud of myself. Yesterday, while at a Vietnamese restaurant in Lethbridge with Linda and friends, I actually consumed a whole big bowl of wonton soup! It was full of vegetables, chicken, noodles, and wontons. Soups go down well because they're liquid, and this meal also has a lot of solid food. The perfect meal for me. And then today, at an Italian restaurant, I ate a half bowl of fettuccine alfredo with chicken. Because of the creamy sauce, it slipped past the inflammation in my throat without too much pain. I usually hate creamy food textures but, in this case, creamy is a good thing.

Recently I've been nibbling on solid foods and sampling a few light soups, but these are the first two actual meals I've eaten. I'm excited. I'm also down to three *Resource 2.0 Tetra Paks* a day. Now I sometimes feel hungry enough to want to eat. Every swallow hurts, but my swallowing coach says I have to suck it up and do it. It helps to drink water to wash the solid foods down. Three weeks ago, I wasn't even drinking water!

My throat is inflamed right where the swallow takes place. Many foods, like those that are acidic or spicy, aggravate that inflammation and cause a stinging sensation. I relieve the stinging with water, but mostly I have to eat bland softer foods. So far, my favourite food is deviled eggs. Among the foods I can't eat are most fruits, avocado and chocolate. They want me eating foods with a lot of cream in them. Gotta learn to love 'em. Linda says it's like weaning a baby off the bottle and introducing new foods. It was easier for her when I was just on the feeding tube. Now she's my meal planner again.

We're jumping into our new Mercedes-Benz Sprinter Cargo Van and heading to Waterton National Park in the Rockies for some RV camping with friends. We love our new van. After hearing my brother-in-law, Gary, talking about the cool guys who kite ski and mountain bike in Hood River Oregon while living in their Sprinter vans, I googled Sprinter vans and was shocked at how expensive the new ones were – $140,000 for a camperized version. But I downloaded a brochure, called a local dealer, and Linda came with me to see one, all the while saying we'll never pay that kind of money. We looked at a few of them and were impressed, except their demos didn't have enough windows. And, of course, the dollars made no sense. Still, the fantasy of traveling around in a self-contained home on wheels intrigued us. Linda asked if they had any used versions. As luck would have it, one had just come into the dealership. It had the perfect window arrangement for Linda. Lots of light. Nice views from all angles. Outfitted with everything a small home would need, including granite countertops. And the price was right – $70,000, bargained down to $64,400. Best of all, it was a 2007 version that had barely been used. Only 34,000 kilometers on it. We went home and scoured the internet for a better deal; there were none in all of Canada or the US. We had the money since I'd just sold my business. So, we bought it. A spur of the moment decision. Now we're nomads. Free to wander. Almost.

I AM FINDING MYSELF OUT OF STEP

We spent two relaxing days in Waterton with our friends, Dave Gillespie and Karen Pumphrey. It was fun hanging out with them and getting a sense of how to live in a small RV. Linda loved it.

We left Waterton and drove for a day to East Barrier Lake, a lovely lake near Kamloops, BC, to visit with my former business coach, Catharine Wright, and her husband, Russ Phillips. They have a beautiful square log home on the lake. We've been here for the past two days. It's very relaxing. Eating, listening to music, playing cards, and just hanging out. We've been for two long walks and I even got to try paddle boarding. I did it without getting wet.

The big news for me is more about eating than travelling. I've been eating enough real food to keep my calorie intake up to 2,000 calories, which means I've been able to cut back to just two *Resource 2.0 Tetra Paks* a day. Each contains 500 calories, and I've successfully replaced four *Tetra Paks* with real food. I've been trying a lot of different foods and my repertoire is expanding. However, eating still hurts because my throat is still inflamed and I have to follow every swallow with a gulp of water. It's an ordeal. It's also probably uncomfortable for Linda to watch as I grimace and make all kinds of gurgling noises, while trying to maneuver the food around and get it down my throat. That said, I manage to eat three actual meals a day.

I can still only eat foods that are soft and/or smooth as they slip down easily. Also, I need foods that are bland as they don't irritate the inflamed area in my throat. Many types of fruit that I'd love to eat are acidic and hurt my throat. Wor Wonton soup has been my best meal so far. I've also eaten quite a few versions of chicken noodle soup. I've eaten a lot of chicken, period. In fact, I can eat any meat, as long as it's soft, cut into small cubes, and covered in sauce. Not huge amounts but enough to keep up the calorie and protein intake. For breakfast, Linda's been making me pancakes or French toast. I was eating them with syrup but have discovered that the taste starts out fine, but ends up leaving a bad aftertaste in my mouth. Sweet is the main taste that has changed for me. Even the fruit I've been eating, like peaches, start out tasting good and then there's a bad aftertaste. I find butter is best on pancakes. It tastes good and helps the food to go down smoothly. I've been eating deviled eggs and they taste good. They're smooth and solid, so they're easy to swallow. I put a lot of salt on them. I like sugar less than before and I appreciate salt more. I'm getting plenty of protein in my meals – lots of eggs and meat. I also get a fair amount of carbs from noodles or bread with butter. I've tried peanut butter, but it sticks just at the swallow point and hurts my throat. I can also eat veggies as long as they are soft and smothered in butter. So, I'm making good progress. It's work, but it has to be done.

I'm stronger now, but I still don't have the energy I used to have. Which is to be expected, I guess. What bothers me more is that I don't seem to be able to think as clearly. Many people who have worked or lived with me have always thought of me as absent-minded. Now it's much worse. Even I think I'm absent minded. I'm constantly finding myself lost or out of step, much more often than ever before. Maybe it's cancer recovery related or maybe it's retirement or maybe it's just getting older, but it frustrates me. Linda's frustrated too. I had thought maybe it's just us living together all day, every day, but now I don't think so. I don't think I'm as sharp as I was. I hope whatever I've lost comes back. Fortunately, I haven't lost my sense of humour so we can at least laugh at my idiocy. This is where I should put in a funny anecdote to illustrate my point, but I can't think of one. See, I am losing it.

But not so much that I don't remember that I have a lot to be thankful for. I'm thankful that I can now eat meals and am getting stronger. I'm also thankful to have good friends to visit, a Sprinter Van to travel in, and Linda to travel through life with. My life is pretty darn good. Even when I'm feeling out of step.

WHEN IS THIS GOING TO BE OVER?

While I'm proud to be making progress with the eating
– three real meals a day and down to one, or at most two
Tetra Paks through my feeding tube – my low energy level
concerns me. We did three hikes in Jasper National Park
this week – Athabasca Falls/ Sunwapta Falls, Maligne
Canyon, and Edith Cavell Meadow. Tourist hikes, each
two to three hours long. These used to be walks, not
hikes, for me.

I felt OK while hiking, but when we got home, I
felt exhausted and, a week later, I still haven't recovered. In fact, Linda is out kayaking right now and I'm
too tired to join her.

But a few days ago, when we were at an open house for the
redevelopment of Dawson Park, a park right near where
we live, I was full of energy and talked to people for three
hours. It was great to see so many of my riding buddies lobbying for the City to not wreck our single-track
mountain bike paths. Many of the guys commented on
how good I looked and how energetic I was. And I was

energetic – then. My energy levels change from day to day and even from hour to hour.

The same is kind of true for my eating. One day I feel very little pain when I swallow and the next day every swallow hurts. My swallowing coach says it's going to be like that for a few months – I will have pain inside my throat and neck region that will come and go. I'm still healing from the radiation. It's not that the pain's so bad; it's just disconcerting. When is this going to be over?

Mostly my eating is getting better. I'm still trying to get off the *Tetra Paks* but not hard enough, so Linda is pushing me. Wor Wonton soup is still my favourite meal but she has also got me eating omelettes, stir-fries, and even meat and potatoes meals. On October 1, I will stop using the feeding tube. Once I've gone for a month on real foods exclusively, they will take the tube out of my stomach.

My weight dropped a pound or two when I went down to two *Tetra Paks* because my calorie intake went down. I weigh 148 pounds now. I need to get 2,500 calories a day with 120 grams of protein to gain weight. Hard to do when it's hard to eat. The good news is that my taste buds seem to be working. I like how food tastes now. The only taste that is distorted is sweetness which, as I've said before, leaves a weird aftertaste. Not too weird to keep me from eating sweet foods, but I don't crave sweets like I used to, and when I do eat something sweet that used to be enjoyable, it's not as satisfying. Treats like ice cream aren't what they used to be. Even fruit doesn't taste as good as I remember. Luckily, I still like most foods, I like to eat, and I sort of look forward to meals. If only it weren't so painful trying to get each swallow of food past the inflammation in my throat.

I often deal with the pain of swallowing by sitting slumped over the kitchen table, holding my forehead in my left hand, with my elbow planted on the table, and focussing on my pain. I feel more comfortable in that posture. It comforts me. Linda says it makes me look depressed and, in fact, it depresses her because I look so despondent. She asked me why I sit that way and I told her, "Habit." I realize now that this is exactly how I used to sit at the family dinner table when I was a pouty, rebellious teenager. Head on my hand, elbow on the table, all wrapped up in myself. Not exactly defiant but clearly, I was not being part of our merry family. My dad hated the way I sat. No wonder he loved my brother best. Linda doesn't let me sit like that anymore. It's too isolating. Suck it up, Kuby, and sit up straight.

My swallowing coach /speech therapist, Anna, showed us some x-rays that allowed us to see what happens when I swallow. I still aspirate. There's a small trickle of water that wants to go toward my windpipe instead of my esophagus. It doesn't make it all the way because I cough or gurgle. Both the coughing and gurgling make me unpleasant to be around at meal time. The cough is my body's natural way of keeping the water from going down the air passage. The gurgling is a technique Anna showed me to clear the water away from my air passage. Anna wants me to learn to eat without any aspiration. Because I have so little of the saliva that would naturally clean my teeth, there's a danger that the liquid going into my lungs will be carrying bacteria that has a chance of causing pneumonia. That could be deadly. At any sign of lung trouble or infection, I would have to go to Emergency.

My teeth are often coated with food after a meal and my mouth is full of gunk. Bits of food collecting in my mouth. So I have to brush, swish, and spit after every meal and at bedtime to clean my teeth and my mouth. It's time-consuming and it's frustrating. We expect the aspiration problem to go away in the coming year and that the saliva will return. That is the hope. It all takes time.

Mostly, I feel and act like I'm cancer-free, but we won't know for sure 'til I get the PET scan on October 11 and see my doctor for the results on October 18. In the meantime, we're getting in the Sprinter van and heading for Saskatchewan for a few days. We are on an informal mission to eventually hit all the national parks in Canada, so the next one is Prince Albert National Park. Then we'll visit our friends, Ernie and Beatrice Meili, in Candle Lake. They're business associates from whom I purchased an educational toy store franchise, Play and Learn Parent Teacher Store, in Edmonton about 40 years ago.

After that, we're off to Winnipeg for my mom's

95th birthday on September 25. Mom is in good health and lives in an independent-living seniors' home. She recently told me that she's been retired for more years than she worked! She has slowed down and doesn't drive or bowl anymore, but she's still quite active. She plays a lot of bridge and makes sure she gets out and about. She recently started going on regular walks. Using her walker for support, she circles the outside of the complex where she lives. It takes about 10 minutes. She says it was slow-going at first and she had to rest often, but now she does it without having to rest. She goes out two or three times a day.

Mom was a mother of six and a registered nurse. When she was in her mid-forties, when my dad's health was failing, she went back to university to upgrade her nursing credentials so she could get work. I used to see her in the hallway at the university heading to her classes while I was skipping mine. She would give me and my friends a bemused smile, chat with us briefly, and then scoot down the hall, carrying her books. She was always considerate and non-judgmental, never one to interfere with anyone else's fun, even her wayward son's. Just one of the reasons so many people love and admire her. My mom rarely has a bad thing to say to, or about, anyone. She just takes things in her stride. I'm blessed to have such a remarkable mother.

I EXPECTED LESS PAIN BY NOW

My energy levels are maybe better and I'm eating a wider variety of foods. However, my throat is more painful, especially in the last few days. This is frustrating. I'd been making such good progress that I expected less pain by now, not more. The last few days have felt like a setback. I know I should be thankful I've come this far, but when you're in pain, it's hard to be thankful.

I still like the same foods – eggs, pancakes or French toast for breakfast, ham and cheese sandwiches and noodle soup for lunch, and meat meals for dinner. I've enjoyed two steak meals and some barbecued ribs. If it's tasty, I seem to be able to eat it even if it hurts to swallow. Which it does at the moment. Every swallow hurts. My throat hurts more than ever, especially on the left side where there's an inflammation that's been driving me crazy. The pain is worse than it used to be and it's been like that for at least a week. Even when I swallow a simple gulp of water, or just a build-up of saliva, there's pain right at the back of the throat where the food begins to go down. So, I try to go for as long as I can without swallowing anything.

When I eat, it's not too pretty. I'm always cringing, making noises, and cradling my head in my hand. Often my food gets caught in my throat right at the inflamed part and will not go down. That really bothers me. I then have to suck it back up into my mouth with a bunch of phlegm and then re-swallow it or spit it into a tissue. Yuk. I know. Sometimes the food just sits there, causing no real pain, but not going down my throat. It's just stuck. That's irritating too. So I suck it up back into my mouth and spit it out into a tissue. I always have a tissue handy. I'm constantly filling up garbage cans with tissues full of gunk.

I'm being graphic about my eating because my intention has always been to record what I'm actually experiencing. I got a comment on my blog from Dr. Walker, my chemotherapy oncologist, saying he was encouraging some of his patients to read it. I was flattered that he would take the time to read my blog and was pleased that it might have something to offer to others with the same cancer.

While I'm describing my aches and pains, I have to add a new one – my jaw. Recently I've been experiencing an almost constant aching on the left side of my jaw, just below my ear. It's a dull ache that sometimes gets sharp. I frequently massage my facial muscles to relieve it. I often have a bit of a headache. I massage my temples and my eyes to try and relieve the ache, and it sort of works but not really. I have to take *Advil* for it. Another reason I'm not jubilant about my progress.

Yesterday, Freda, a friend of my mom's and a regular commenter on my blog, came to visit us at my mom's place in Winnipeg. Freda had tongue cancer 10 years ago and her experience was much more frustrating than mine. She had to use a feeding tube for 54 weeks and had to have surgery to open her throat so she could eat again. I don't know if this was due to the nature of her cancer, or its location in her throat, or if treatments have improved since she had her cancer. Maybe all three. Now she's doing well. Full of energy and enthusiasm for life. Baked me a delicious cake. She suggested that for my throat pain I should try gargling with salt water and, surprisingly, it has helped a lot. It takes some of the pain away.

We've been travelling in the Sprinter for the past ten days. Sightseeing and hiking at Waskesiu in Prince Albert National Park was nice. The leaves were a lovely mix of yellow, red, and green. I took a ton of pictures. Staying with the Meilis at their cabin at Candle Lake was interesting and inspiring. I was impressed by all the hiking, biking and kayaking trips and other traveling that they'd done since retiring at 55. They're now 72 and in great health. Looks like we retired too late. Oh well.

Ernie got me started in my own business when I was 31. I was a hotshot sales rep for a competing company, selling school supplies and teaching aids to elementary schools. When Ernie offered me a Play and Learn Parent Teacher Store franchise, I took it on with a friend, Bill Lawrence. It was a retail and mail order business that lasted quite a few years. We operated the retail store in Edmonton and I was the sales rep for Ernie's Play and Learn catalogue/mail order business, selling directly to schools. That business morphed into my own company selling playground equipment – PlayWorks, Inc., the company I grew to 15 employees and just recently sold. I'd always been a good salesperson and became even more focussed when I started selling playground equipment. Designing playgrounds and selling playground equipment was my calling, and I have Ernie to thank for helping me find it. PlayWorks, Inc. also provided me with a great way to make a living. I've been blessed.

Ernie took us on a beautiful hike at Candle Lake and introduced us to pickleball later in the afternoon. Pickleball seems like a great sport for seniors. Hey, we're now retired seniors. Beatrice and Ernie treated us to some great meals and taught us the card game, Wizard. I guess playing cards is another retirement activity we can enjoy.

After leaving the Meilis, we drove to Riding Mountain National Park where we did some more hiking – usually about four to five kilometers in length for about an hour and a half at a time.

Celebrating Mom's 95th birthday was fun, although when I walked through her seniors' home, I felt like I fit right in. I have grey hair, I'm skinny and frail, and I move slowly. All I was missing was a walker.

My sister D-Anne, who lives in Winnipeg, my brother Sandy from Abbotsford, BC, and my sister Shenta from Spruce Grove, Alberta were also there for the occasion. We all piled into the Sprinter van and drove to Grand Beach, a huge sandy beach on Lake Winnipeg with big sand dunes. It was cold, rainy, and very windy, but we had fun being together. D-Anne surprised us by stripping down to a bathing suit and going for a swim in the big waves. Brrrrr!

Later, we drove back to Winnipeg, and all went to The Keg for steak dinner with Shirley, one of mom's best friends. When we got home, my mom was exhausted and fell asleep in her chair. She'd recovered by morning though, and seemed happy with her special day. Later on, she left us to go play with one of her regular bridge groups. At 95, she often wins.

We leave tomorrow for Saskatoon for a quick visit with Allie, the PlayWorks sales rep in Saskatoon, and her husband, Noah. I intend to photograph some of her better playgrounds when we're there. Photographing playgrounds was one of the fun things I always liked doing when I was working. We'll try to be back to Edmonton in time for Gary Arnold's annual birthday bonfire party.

Progress on the recovery front. I just found out that I don't have to see my swallowing coach and dietician on a regular basis any more. Instead, I will join a support group for throat cancer patients who are all using a feeding tube.

They meet every couple of weeks. I'll be going to my first meeting when I get back.

We're going out for supper tonight with friends from Winnipeg – Richard Stecenko and his wife, Lorna, with Ken and Sandra Friesen. I'm worried that I won't be able to enjoy the gourmet meal that Richard is preparing for us, but I'm sure Linda will. And I'll have fun, anyway. Earlier we were invited to dinner with an old friend from high school, Eric Sawyer and his wife Joanie. Eric built a big insurance practice in Winnipeg and we had fun comparing notes on how lucky we've been and how hard we worked to create that luck. I've been blessed with good friends.

While visiting in my mom's seniors' residence, I connected with Diane Proux, who is my age and was a classmate in high school. She's in a seniors' home because she suffers from Alzheimer's. Too young to be in a seniors' home for sure, but when I talked to her, she was youthful, sharp, clear-minded, and fun to chat with. She was a school teacher and has lived a great life. Now she's clearly happy to be in a home where she has others to rely on when she needs support. She told me how the staff and residents have supported her, and how every morning her sister helps her write a plan to follow for that day and calls later in the day to see if she's following it. She seems to have a lot going on. Diane was happy and very thankful. I was very impressed with her, and her sister.

It was also flattering to learn that Diane had had a big crush on me when we were in high school. Too bad she told me 55 years too late. She was someone I knew and liked but we never ran in the same circles. I had no idea she had a crush on me. I told her I was flattered but that I'd spent my high school years mooning after another girl. One who barely knew I liked her. Nice to know that such a smart girl was quietly attracted to me when I was young and foolish.

I'M NOT GETTING BETTER

The aching in my jaw and my headaches are worse. The inflammation on the left side of my throat is worse, to the point where I've quit trying to eat meals. My pain in my jaw and the related headaches started about a week ago and are getting harder to deal with. Before I could sort of massage them away, then I used *Advil*, then *Advil Extra Strength*, and now I'm having to use liquid morphine to deal with the pain.

The pain is not specific to one spot. I feel it along my jaw and, to a lesser degree, all along the bones of my face and eyes. It's sometimes quite severe in my temples and on the side of my head, up where my jaw bones meet my right ear. That would suggest an earache, but it seems different from earaches I've had. I also don't think it's a toothache because it doesn't seem related to my teeth. But now and then I get a random shot of pain from my back teeth to my ear, so who knows?

The inflammation in my throat also doesn't seem to be related; it feels like a different issue. The right side of my face is inflamed, so inflamed that I don't want food to touch it. On Friday, I had to quit eating halfway through lunch and again at supper. So I ate through my feeding tube. I used the feeding tube for all three meals on Saturday and also drank two *Ensures*. That gave me about 2,100 calories, I had trouble eating all last week and noticed that when we got home from Manitoba I'd lost weight. I started the trip about 13 days ago at 149 pounds and am now down to 144 pounds. People tell me I look OK, but at 144 pounds, I'm skinny and have no muscle.

When I'm in pain, I'm grumpy. I also become sort of non-functional as I focus on my pain relief and forget to take care of ordinary duties. You can imagine how this is going down with Linda. She's understanding, but it's hard on her. I think she misses the old me. The new me doesn't want to talk much because talking hurts my throat and I'm often not in a good mood. There's a lot of silence between us right now.

We spent a good Sunday morning together though. It's nice to be home after almost two weeks of living in the Sprinter van. The van is nice to travel in, but home is home. Good to be back in my comfortable easy chair. The one by the window that used to be Linda's favourite spot in the house before I took it over. The cancer card always used to win, but I think it's losing its power over Linda. She wants her chair back.

I'VE GOT THRUSH

The pain I've been experiencing over the past week is now being attributed to a yeast infection called thrush. In the past, the doctors and nurses had mentioned thrush as something that is common for tongue and throat cancer patients. Now I've got it. The main indicator of thrush is white foamy saliva on the tongue. I didn't have that symptom, but my nurse practitioner told us that the pain often comes before the white stuff. Sure enough, yesterday the white stuff appeared. The doctor prescribed nystatin, an anti-fungal medication. It's a thick sweet mouthwash that I swish and swallow three times a day for ten days. The idea is to coat the affected areas with the nystatin. That sounded reassuring until I discovered that the nystatin aggravates the exact area on my tongue and the back of my throat that hurts the most. Just swallowing the medication is agony.

So, to kill the pain, they gave me a liquid morphine prescription. I take it every three or four hours, a half hour before I take the nystatin. Unfortunately, the morphine is not strong enough to kill the pain from the mouthwash on my tongue and throat. Now I can feel the thrush pain with every swallow. The pain has become so acute that I can no longer eat. I'm now taking all of my meals through the feeding tube. This is a setback to my goal of being able to feed myself enough food that I can have the feeding tube removed from my stomach.

Unfortunately, that isn't my only challenge. I'm still experiencing the pain in my left jaw bone, especially where it meets the ear. It's like an earache or a toothache, but according to the nurse practitioner, it's neither. I've been told that it's not uncommon for throat and tongue cancer patients to experience jaw bone pain like this at around three to six months after the radiation treatments.

It's also very likely that the pain from the thrush is triggering the pain in my facial bones. I can also feel the pain along my cheek bones and in my temples along the side of my head. Massage and deep breathing help bring some relief but do not get rid of it. The liquid morphine dulls the pain but it's still always there. When the morphine wears off, it wears off suddenly, and the pain comes back with a vengeance. So, I hurry to take another hit to get some relief.

I'm not battling cancer. What I'm battling is the impact of the radiation that we hope has killed the cancer. As I've said, I go for my PET scan on Tuesday, October 11, and will then meet my doctor on October 18 for the results. That is when I expect the doctor to declare me cancer-free. I hope I'll be "thrush-free" too.

Then I will really feel like celebrating.

LESSONS LEARNED:
I AM READY FOR THIS
LET THE HEALING BEGIN

- Focus on getting better
- Make lists and follow them
- Track your progress
- Be grateful and thankful
- Be patient: recovery can be slow
- Life is good
- Step, step, step: one foot in front of the other
- Don't ever smoke. If you do, now is the time to quit.
- Go for walks or do yoga when you are too tired to exercise
- Share your journal; turn "me time" into "we time".
- Family and friends matter so much

LINDA'S CAREGIVER NOTES:

When John stopped talking, the light went out of our relationship. It was another loss of who we'd been and what we'd had. We were going through enormous changes – the cancer, selling the business, suddenly being together 24/7 – and there was no easy way to discuss it.

As he has explained, we were talkers. A one-sided conversation is very unsatisfactory. We were both on edge. John was impatient that the recovery was taking too long, and I was impatient with his impatience!

Our kayaking adventure was an analogy of what we were going through. Life had been sunny and suddenly we were hit by a storm called cancer. We both had to hold on to the truth that "this too will pass." We were in it together and just had to keep paddling. At the time, it was hard to imagine the cancer storm ever ending, but we had to keep on paddling anyway.

There is a balance to be struck between being supportive and nagging. It was not always easy for me to achieve that balance. I wanted to help but there wasn't much I could do to make John comfortable. I'm sure I was irritating or maybe just irritated that I couldn't fix things.

I did miss the old John. I knew we loved each other, and we could eventually get our old relationship back. I also knew from his blog that he recognized the stress that I was feeling. We were both feeling guilty, even though we both knew that guilt was a useless emotion to carry.

I didn't feel as though I was doing much for John besides worrying about him, which wasn't helpful. So when my kids came to visit, it was an opportunity to take a mental health break. I also had to learn to trust that he would be OK being left with his son, Michael, for a few days. Getting out of the house for walks, exercise, and trips helped change my focus. It was good for both John and me.

CANCER-FREE:

I STILL FEEL LIKE SHIT

PET SCAN RESULTS – GOOD NEWS AND BAD NEWS

My Doctor called today with the PET Scan results. First the good news. The radiation treatments have eliminated all of the cancer. The primary cancer on my tongue is gone and my lymph nodes are clear. Now the bad news. The PET scan shows two new spots on my lungs. They could be cancerous, the doctor thinks it's inflammation, but no one knows for sure. Cancer spreading from my throat to my lungs would be unusual, especially since HPV cancer doesn't spread. Also, since radiation has killed the cancer in my throat, it should have also killed any cancer spreading to my lungs.

Inflammation seems more likely. Probably caused by bacteria in food that has gone down my windpipe. My doctor and my swallowing coach have both been concerned about this because I aspirate when I swallow. These spots could be confirmation that food and liquids that should go down my esophagus are getting into my lungs.

There are two approaches we can take. We can biopsy

the two spots to determine if they are cancerous. Or, we can wait six weeks for the CT scan to see if they've grown or shrunk. If they've shrunk, it's inflammation. If they've grown, it's probably cancer. Cancer doesn't get smaller. On the doctor's recommendation, we're waiting for the CT scan six weeks from now and aren't thinking about it until then. Except when we can't help thinking about it.

Meanwhile, the thrush symptoms remain. There's still white foam on my tongue and throat and the inflammation at the base and side of my tongue is still painful. It bothers me when I talk and every time I swallow. While the thrush itself causes pain in the inflamed area, the more serious pain is in my facial muscles and bones, which the doctors think is being triggered by the thrush. It feels like a toothache without a specific aching tooth. It also feels like an earache except the pain is not specific to my ear. I feel it in my jaw bones and cheek bones, and along my eye sockets and temples. I'm managing the pain with liquid morphine, but it's taking progressively more morphine to keep the pain under control. Because of the pain in my mouth, I'm still eating from my feeding tube exclusively. This is a serious setback to my recovery

Despite my cancer-free diagnosis, I don't feel like I am progressing. The cancer battle may be over and done with, but the battle against thrush and the pain in my face rages on. It drowns out any satisfaction I may feel that the cancer is gone. I'm trying to see the glass as 90% full, not just half full, but positive thinking is almost impossible when you're in pain.

I'm taking Nystatin and acidophilous to get rid of the thrush. The morphine can kill the pain for an hour and half or longer. It's unpredictable. When the pain comes back, it comes back with a vengeance, and I need another dose quickly. I try to time the new dose so that it kicks in before the last one wears off. It takes 20 minutes for the new morphine to kick in. If I time it wrong and don't take it early enough, I writhe in pain before the new dose eventually brings relief. This happens frequently because I never know precisely when the last dose will wear off. It can work for as little as an hour and a half or as long as three hours. I often get the timing wrong and can find myself in severe pain for 15 or 20 minutes, which feels like an eternity.

When I'm gripped by that pain, I will do almost anything to stop it, but all that's available to me is massaging my temples and doing deep breathing. It's hard to be patient and trust the morphine, but it always kicks in eventually. Slow deep breathing, slow deep breathing.

I find that cannabis oil, or *Phoenix Tears*, supports the morphine and extends the pain-free period. I've also been using it to put me to sleep at night and I find it also makes me sleep in longer. I wake up in the morning feeling groggy and a little stoned, but I've slept well. I really don't like feeling stoned during the day, but I'm tempted to take *Phoenix Tears* more often and see what happens. It's choosing a bit of mental confusion over a lot of physical pain. Not a hard choice to make.

Maybe being stoned is the best way to follow the last 30 days of the Dump Trump Parade. I have found it difficult to concentrate lately so I'm watching a lot of TV. Thank God for sports or I'd be watching nothing but "The Donald." The Oilers' hockey season started with a win and they look like they could make the playoffs this year. The Blue Jays are still in the game. I have them to cheer for. And hearing that Bob Dylan was being awarded the Nobel Prize for Literature took my mind off the Trump takeover, briefly.

Snowboarding season starts on November 10 in the Rockies. I wonder how ready I'll be.

As long as there is a chance that there is cancer in my lungs, I'm going to feel a bit nervous. Six weeks will be a long wait. Bring on the *Phoenix Tears*.

SLOW TO NO PROGRESS

No real change. I still feel shitty and I'm not sure what to write about any more. It's been ten days since I've written anything. Part of me doesn't want to recount this litany of irritants and issues I'm dealing with because they're a boring read and why would anyone be interested? Another part of me says I should continue to document how I'm actually experiencing this crazy cancer adventure. Just capture what it is, boring or not. I've decided to go that route.

Yes, this account is a litany of the aches, pains, irritants and frustrations that make up my day. I hope I don't come across as giving up. I'm not. I'm just frustrated with my lack of progress.

I saw the doctor again last Tuesday. Linda and I watched the screen as he put the scope down my nostril and into my throat. The little camera showed us a patch of white foam on the left side of my throat, which seems to be inflammation from the thrush. Other than that, everything looked very healthy.

The cancer has gone. The doctor has assured us that those spots on my lungs are not likely cancerous and he's not worried. We will know for sure in five weeks.

Unfortunately, the yeast infection, or thrush, is not getting any better. I still have pain on the left side at the back of my tongue, which is covered with foamy white spots. The nystatin hasn't cleared it up, so I have a prescription for a stronger drug, fluconazole. I hope it works.

The inflammation on my tongue makes it painful to eat. Thanks to the thrush, I'm still only eating through my feeding tube and now weigh between 144 and 146 pounds. Not good. I also have a bad taste in my mouth most of the time. A minor irritation, yes, but I have it, and it's not pleasant. I am still dealing with build-ups of phlegm from my nose and throat, and frequently have to spit into the sink or into a tissue to get rid of it. The phlegm is not as bad as it used to be, but it hasn't gone away. It's still a problem.

The greater concern is the unrelenting pain in my facial muscles and bones. I'm managing the pain by taking morphine pills every couple of hours. Self-massage and deep breathing also help, but without the morphine I would be in constant agony. How could anyone ever get through this without morphine? I thank God for morphine, but there's a downside. I'm in a morphine fog. My thinking is muddled, I lose track of time, I can't remember what I've done from one moment to the next, and I get flustered easily. Normal life is hard to manage. My life doesn't flow as easily. I want my brain back.

I also feel tired a lot of the time. I experience it as a heaviness across the back of my neck and shoulders. Deep breathing and relaxation exercises help, but sometimes I feel like I could be doing them all day long. I've been sleeping a lot. I don't know if it's the morphine or the cannabis oil I've been taking at bedtime, but I'm sometimes sleeping in until late in the morning. Plus I take naps. Yes, I know, sleeping is therapeutic, but all of this sleep doesn't feel beneficial.

In general, I don't feel good about myself. I often feel out of sorts and I don't seem to have the energy or the discipline to take advantage of all the free time I have. Not only am I not doing anything productive, I'm also not doing the healthy and relaxing things that would help in my recovery. I don't even go for walks. I've only gone on one walk since we got back from Winnipeg.

I still read and listen to music, but not nearly as much. I haven't read a new book in two months. I find it hard to do much of anything. For instance, writing about my cancer adventure used to be easy, but now it's hard, so I'm not writing as much either.

What do I do with my time? Too much Facebook, too much web surfing, and too much Donald Trump, that's what. Thank God for hockey games. Can you believe the

Edmonton Oilers are number one in the league after six games?

It doesn't take a genius to figure out I'm not good company for Linda these days. I often find it hard to talk because of the throat pain. Even worse, I find I'm not sharp enough to stay on top of what's going on, so I tend to not take part in normal daily conversation like I used to. I frequently feel out of step, so sometimes I don't try to keep up. To make matters worse, Linda is using hearing aids and sometimes she doesn't put them in. Besides, my voice is deeper and quieter now, which makes it harder for her to hear me properly at the best of times, so I often have to repeat myself. It's a strain for me to talk, which makes things even more frustrating. I end up regretting having started any light conversation because what starts out as a simple observation or question ends up becoming way too complicated.

As a result, our conversations are shorter and not as deep. The communication barriers also throw off my comic timing, so we don't banter with each other like we used to. It's a strain on our relationship for sure, but Linda is understanding and we're adapting.

The new thrush medication and the morphine both have the potential to upset my stomach so I sometimes feel waves of nausea. Even while writing this, I've felt nausea coming on and have had to run to the toilet to throw up. I just emptied my stomach of the last tetra pack of

Resource 2.0 into the sink. White vomit. How's that for a visual? Yuk. Interesting that before I threw up, I'd been writing all these negative thoughts. Maybe they were reflecting how I was feeling physically. Maybe they made me want to puke.

I've since had a long recovery nap and am feeling rejuvenated. As I finish writing this after an evening of watching TV, I feel better. It's hard to pin down how I'm feeling because it's constantly changing.

Many of my cancer buddies have recommended various medications for getting rid of thrush, including honey concoctions. Someone even gave me the rest of the mouthwash he'd been prescribed for thrush when he had it. I haven't tried any special remedies yet, but I bought some acidophilous pills that someone had suggested. It's a probiotic, similar to what's found in yogurt, which I dislike eating because it's too soft and gooey.

WORST NIGHT OF MY LIFE

The day after my last writing, my facial pain suddenly disappeared and the thrush vanished. Maybe it was the new drug or maybe the probiotics. I still feel weak and out of sorts, but with the facial pain gone, I feel more optimistic. Progress is being made. No facial pain means I didn't need the morphine anymore, so I quit taking it. Just stopped taking the 10 ml I'd been taking every two hours for couple of weeks. Cold turkey.

Big mistake! I'm an educated person and should have known better. Even Linda didn't know. We both thought I wasn't taking enough morphine, or for long enough, to worry about withdrawal effects. We didn't even discuss it. We even mentioned being two days morphine-free to our nurse practitioner at Tuesday's support group session. No one said anything to us about going off morphine too fast.

I sure got a taste of just how bad it can be. Bad.

According to what Linda just read on-line, "withdrawal symptoms start 36 hours after you stop taking morphine." In my case that was true. It started just before bed time. You know how, when you've been up drinking all night and you throw up before hitting the bed, you can at least count on getting a long night's sleep. Not this time. I started vomiting, throwing up, hurling, puking, whatever you want to call it. It didn't matter that there was nothing in my stomach to puke up. Sharp convulsions, dry retching, and dry heaves continued long after my stomach was empty. Once I started throwing up, it kept coming and coming and coming with only short rests in between. It was unrelenting.

After each attack, I would lie there, trying to calm down, trying to practice my deep breathing. Mostly I tossed from side to side and massaged my muscles trying to get comfortable. Now and then, I would fall asleep only to wake up feeling like I was about to vomit and would have to quickly lean over the edge of the bed and hurl into the bucket again. I was getting sleep in maybe 15-minute intervals. The pattern just kept repeating itself, no relief. My stomach was empty after the first few attacks, so mostly I was dry retching. Violent dry retches that hurt. My stomach was searching for something to throw up. I started to drink water, which helped. It didn't hurt as much and the experience was more "rewarding." If you can call vomiting black bile rewarding.

Linda stayed up with me all night trying to comfort me. There wasn't much she could do other than be there. Which I appreciated.

The puking was only part of the experience. There were chills and sweats, and body aches and pains, but fortunately none of that was very severe. I didn't seem to have a high temperature either. I reminded myself that this could all be so much worse. Note to self: Never become a drug addict.

Once I finished retching, I couldn't lie there comfortably. I couldn't find a way to lie in my bed that didn't aggravate the muscle pain in my chest and stomach caused by all the dry heaves. Eventually, at around 6 AM, we pumped my stomach full of *Resource 2.0* so I would have something to puke up; we hoped that maybe, just maybe, some food would calm my stomach down. It did make the vomiting events less frequent. That was a blessing.

Linda eventually went to sleep. I kept right on puking, with longer and longer periods in between. By mid-morning, I'd slept soundly for an hour or two. When we got up at around noon, our first step was to call the doctor who, of course, said, "No, no, no, you can't quit morphine cold turkey like that!"

Morphine withdrawal? Really? That had never occurred to us, but we were relieved to know there was an explanation.

He gave us a general guideline that we followed. I got back on the morphine in gradually reduced amounts. I felt weak and tired all day yesterday. The nausea didn't go away immediately and there was still some hurling, but taking more morphine helped.

In the afternoon, as I was walking to our bedroom, my cell phone rang and I picked it up. It was Pat, a sales rep from PlayWorks. After saying "Hi, Pat," I realized that I was about to puke, so I asked him to wait. Which he did. I filled the bucket beside my bed and then we chatted. Gross! Luckily, Pat used to be a paramedic, so he could handle it.

By the time the day was over and the Oilers had beaten Alexander Ovechkin and the Washington Capitals, I was feeling much improved. No doubt because I was back on morphine again. I took a sleeping pill before bed and I think it helped. I slept well. No "events."

JOY? FEEL IT WHEN YOU CAN

I woke up this morning and realized I was feeling no nausea, no facial pain, no pain in my throat (well, not much), no real discomfort anywhere. What I felt was... joy. Not a word I use a lot. But the room was bright, my bed was warm, Linda was beside me sleeping, and I wasn't in any pain. I felt joyful. So I lay in bed and let myself feel the joy for a while. Get it while you can, Kuby. This too will pass.

We now have a program of pills that includes morphine in decreasing amounts, an anti- nausea pill, and a pill to get rid of the thrush. There are still a few remnants of white foam on my tongue, but the pain in my throat has receded. My swallowing isn't "normal" yet, but it also doesn't hurt like it used to.

After the last couple of days, I've been feeling relieved to just be sitting here in my big chair typing and not feeling nauseous or sick. But no rest for the wicked – I have to do more than luxuriate my way to health. I have to get back to actually eating again. A month ago, I'd been eating almost all of my meals, but since getting the thrush, I've been getting all of my food through the feeding tube. Now that the thrush is gone, it's time to get back in the saddle. Besides, I've been losing weight. I had been at 146 to 148 pounds for a month, down from my normal 165. Today I hit the scale at 136 pounds. Yes, 136. I've lost 30 pounds. When anyone tells me I'm "looking good," I know they're lying. I look gaunt.

The last time I weighed 136 pounds, I was 19 years old and playing varsity hockey for the University of Winnipeg Wesmen. I remember the coach announcing at our first weigh-in that I was 30 pounds lighter than the next lightest guy on the team. Even Gretzky weighed 165 pounds. I centred the second line, but didn't play much that season because I was injured most of the time. Too small to be playing against the big boys.

Speaking of playing with the big boys. If I ever want to ride with the F'n Riders again, I have to do a lot of work to get back to being as strong as them. I wasn't fat when I weighed 165 pounds, so most of the 30 pounds I've lost must be muscle. Being able to ride hard on a mountain bike for two or three hours seems a long way off, but it's a worthy goal.

The first step is to go for more walks with Linda. And do yoga. And then resistance training with light weights. I have a fat bike, so I can do some riding in the snow this winter. Snowboarding season starts in mid-November. I hope I'm ready for that. I have to progress slowly but I do have to progress. Remember, "No quit in me."

I sound like a man ready to live again. A big improvement over the last few days.

IT'S UGLY BUT IT'S PROGRESS

Nothing dramatic is happening. It's just slow, steady, boring progress. My thrush has gone. My facial pain has gone. I'm slowly weaning myself off the morphine. I don't have enough pain to warrant being on it, but the doctor is making sure I get off the stuff gradually. I'm down to about a third of the morphine I'd been taking before.

I still have the pain in my throat. At my doctor's visit today, he said that the spot where the thrush was causing the pain was where I got the heaviest dose of radiation. It will take a long time to fully heal – anywhere from two to six months. He used the scope again, and we saw images of my throat. It was very healthy-looking, except for one inflamed patch on the left side of my throat.

That's the only place where I feel pain now. As long as I tilt my head and channel the food or water along the right side I can swallow without too much pain. I look awkward holding my head parallel to the table as I eat, but at least I'm eating. I still have to gurgle as I swallow, to keep the food from going down my windpipe.

It's ugly, but it's progress. Having just started eating by mouth a few days ago, I don't eat enough to keep my weight up, so I'm also downing three *Tetra Paks* of *Resource 2.0* through the feeding tube. I still need to go for a month without using the feeding tube before they'll take it out of my stomach. My goal is to have it out in December, which means that over the next month, I need to be eating three meals a day and progressively gaining weight. This morning, I ate deviled eggs for breakfast along with yogurt and a cup of berries (frozen berries are my treat these days), and tonight I had wor wonton soup.

I now weigh 142 pounds – up from the puny 136. Nonetheless, I look gaunt, I feel weak, and I tire very easily during a walk. I even get tired doing chores around the house. (Not that I do much work around the house, or ever did). After any exertion, I recover slowly and have to nap or rest. Even if we just go for a short drive to get out of the house for a while, I have to rest when we get back.

So I'm not doing much. I'm just sitting around watching the Oilers and the Trump news. Trying to read but it's hard to concentrate. Still a bit brain dead.

Linda has been great at looking after me but she decided a couple of days ago that, since I'm on the mend, she can take a break. She drove down to Lethbridge a couple of days ago to visit her mother. Good for her. She deserves a break from me. I'll be OK on my own for a week. And my son Mike, who lives in the basement suite, is here.

Even though I'm getting better, I'm frustratingly slow at everything. I'm still more scatterbrained and forgetful than ever. It's frustrating for Linda and I sympathize. Frankly, it's frustrating for me too. We laugh about it, but it's no laughing matter. I can hold a conversation for a while and I can be fairly social, but it doesn't take much to wear me out. Any setback weakens me. I worry that I'll never get my old self back.

The tired feeling pervades my neck and shoulder muscles, so I take naps and do yoga exercises. Deep breathing helps too. Linda and I have continued to walk, and sometimes I can go for an hour or so, but then I take an hour to fully recover. My doctor says there's good evidence that exercise speeds recovery, so he encourages me to exercise but not to overdo it. I struggle with finding that balance. Yesterday, I did a resistance workout with light weights and felt good, but today I'm taking a complete rest. Tomorrow I'll go for a walk again.

Now that the thrush pain has gone I am supposed to get back on my "care for my teeth" regime. This involves a fluoride treatment once a day as well as brushing and flossing three times a day. The fluoride hurt my mouth when I had the thrush, but now I have canker sores that hurt when I use the fluoride. If it's not one thing, it's another. Baking soda seems to help get rid of the canker sores.

While I'm on a roll and doing all of this complaining, let me add that I also have a bad taste in my mouth all the time. A taste that just won't go away. I'm sure my breath is no prize either. Maybe it's from the morphine or maybe it's left over from the thrush. It could also be from four months of feeding myself through a feeding tube. To pile on another complaint, I had no issues with the feeding tube before, but recently I have felt bloated, especially during the evening and later at night. Not that I throw up; I just have an unsettled stomach. I burp a lot to relieve the pressure. Gross.

I have to remember that I've committed to writing about what is happening, not about what might be entertaining. If I feel like shit, I have to write about it. You can see why Linda had to go see her Mom. I'm not in serious pain anymore; I'm just uncomfortable and no fun to be around. I see what I've written here, and it looks like whining. Oh, well. Whining is what I'm doing, and I deserve the opportunity to do it.

One thing I've learned about this slow recovery is that no matter what's happening today, it will be different tomorrow. From what I can tell, I am on a good trajectory, so likely it will be better different, not worse different. Maybe I've been a little too impatient.

Is there anything entertaining, or at least upbeat, to write about? We're staying home for Christmas. And we're going to Costa Rica for most of January and February.

We're looking forward to hanging out with Lorna and George. They recently moved to Costa Rica from Atlanta, Georgia. I accuse them of being among the first to escape the US before it all falls apart under Trump. Prescient of me, since I said that before the election results.

My friend Antoine told me about a beach in Costa Rica, near a town called Samara, where the waves are perfect for beginning surfers. So perfect that even children and old men can learn how to surf. Predictable waves, shallow water. I can't wait to give it a go. Since Linda wants sunshine and flowers in the winter, Costa Rica style, I have to find a new sport to replace snowboarding. Maybe surfing will be it.

In the meantime, I can't wait 'til the snow gets here so I can get on my snowboard again. I don't think it'll be too strenuous as long as I don't push myself. Patience, Kuby, patience.

MY FIRST SUPPORT GROUP

We were at the Cross Cancer Institute recently. Our first visit of the day was with my swallowing coach, Anna. She's actually a speech pathologist, but her job is to make sure throat cancer patients don't lose their ability to swallow. I'm not one of her better patients. I aspirate as I swallow. Water and bits of food go down my windpipe and she's concerned. The worry is that bacteria in the food can cause infection in the lungs, which can lead to pneumonia.

The last CT scan showed small spots in my lungs, which we hope will have gone away by now. It could be an infection due to aspirated food. It could also be another cancer, but we're fairly sure it isn't. We won't actually know until my next CT scan in a couple of weeks.

She tested my swallow by graphing the motions on a chart to monitor the patterns. She was pleased with my progress but continues to be concerned. I still aspirate, but not as badly as before. She warned me that I have to do my exercises or my swallowing may not improve. If I leave it too long, the throat will get rigid and won't get better, ever.

to cure as some other cancers, but, because of where the cancer is and because of the pervasive effects of radiation treatments on the rest of your body and on your life, the extra care is warranted. The psychologist explained that the effects of oral cancer and recovery from radiation and/or surgery are varied and that many of the losses a person suffers have a major impact, not just on the patient's health but on their total sense of well-being.

Weight loss, strength loss, exhaustion, pain, swallowing problems, loss of appetite, taste bud changes, dry mouth, choking, mucus management issues, mouth sores, foul tastes, nausea, vomiting, burning sensations, constipation, inability to talk, facial changes, turkey neck, sleep deprivation, fear, memory loss, brain fog, and concentration problems. Quite a list. Any one of these issues would be hard to deal with but for people with tongue/throat cancer, the issues travel in packs and just keep on coming and coming and coming. You get one thing under control and all of a sudden another appears, or it comes back a month later. Experiencing several of them at the same time has a compounding effect.

Most people's social life revolves around eating and drinking; we're always sharing meals or drinks of some sort. But throat cancer patients are cut off from the pleasures of eating and the social life that goes with them. Add that to the list of physical stuff we have to deal with. Not a walk on the beach.

Life is hard but it's much harder when you have tongue cancer.

I'm now committed to doing 30 repetitions of three different swallow exercises a day. Like every other program that's good for you – easy to do, even easier to not do.

After meeting with Anna, we went to my first head and neck cancer support group with a few other patients with tongue or throat cancer. The group meets once a week with a nurse practitioner, speech pathologist, nutritionist, psychologist, and other support people from the Cross. The numbers vary but there are generally between six and 12 of us, depending on the day.

It's interesting to see how individual participants, who are all finished with their radiation, struggle with related but not identical issues. We've all had similar cancers, but in slightly different locations in the throat and tongue. Because the radiation hits each person differently and we all react differently, none of us has the same experience as anyone else. But, the similarities are there and the struggle to stay on top of it all is comparable. It's interesting to share our stories. I find it therapeutic and others shared that same sentiment in the group yesterday. It's always good to be in the supportive company of others who are experiencing some of the same shit you're going through. Anna told us that the Cross Cancer Institute puts more resources, people, money, and time into patients recovering from head and neck cancer than they do for any other cancer patient group. This is because, generally, our cancer is the hardest cancer to recover from. It is rarely a fatal cancer, and maybe it's not as painful or impossible

LESSONS LEARNED:
I STILL FEEL LIKE SHIT

- Pain killers are amazing; but be very careful.
- Communication errors happen when assumptions are made. Do not assume.
- Be forgiving when errors occur.
- Illness and weakness strain even the best relationships
- As good as it is, or as bad it feels, this too will pass.
- Nurture your recovery. Slow but steady.
- Sharing your story in regular patient support group meetings has healing power.
- Every cancer is different; and every patient experiences their cancer differently.
- Any health-related loss will be accompanied by a weakened sense of wellbeing.

LINDA'S CAREGIVER NOTES:

Cancer and cancer recovery changed our relationship. It is hard to say what did it but there were many stresses. Pain creates a grumpy guy who is not pleasant to be around. His "brain fog" was also very frustrating for both of us.

I took time for myself. I went for walks, visited my mother in Lethbridge, and enjoyed time outdoors. We were very lucky to live in the river valley where I could escape into nature. Also, John was sick in the spring and summer, so it was easy to get outdoors.

The time of year was a bonus. Several times a week from late May into the fall, we drove to John's appointments at the Cross Cancer Institute along a route beside the North Saskatchewan River. The road was lined with hanging pots overflowing with flowers that the City of Edmonton planted every Spring. It was a lovely drive and it lifted my spirits every time. I shudder to think what it would have been like in the winter.

It was also a blessing to be in a support group. We received tips from other patients and their spouses and we experienced the comradery of fellow travellers. It helped to be with a group of people who could relate to what we were going through. Some were further along in their recovery, so we could see that life improved with time.

INTEGRATION:

NORMAL IS NOT WHAT
IT USED TO BE

THE NEW PERSON I'VE BECOME

One of the first things I noticed when radiation treatments were over was a disruption in our social life. No more dining out with Linda. No more dinners with friends. No more beers with my biking buddies.

Having been a physically active person, the possibility of that aspect of my life being diminished or nonexistent scares me. It would be a real personal loss. A significant loss of identity. I was a mountain biker. Now I'm not really. I may be again, but I fear that I may not. It's a certainty that it'll be hard to get my base fitness level back. Tough sledding as they say.

There's also the challenge of dealing with the new person I've become. I'm not the person I was in many ways, and I'm not sure I'll ever be that guy again.

It's also been hard on our marriage. Thank God I'm with Linda, who's so wise and understanding. But it's been hard on her too. She doesn't have the life she used to have. We've both lost something from my tongue cancer.

I've lost, she's lost, and together we've lost. Not the end of the world, we will endure, but still...it's hard.

Our support group has been helpful. The team of specialists at our meetings are well aware of the challenges tongue cancer brings; that alone is a big help to all participants. Sharing our experience in a supportive environment and in the company of fellow patients, who offer their own wisdom and experience, and medical specialists, who can answer our individual questions, is invaluable. I'm beyond grateful for it. Each person in the group gets as much time as needed to talk about what's happening for him or her physically and emotionally. Our facilitator makes sure we're all heard and that each of us participates.

There's also a comprehensive, free program at the University of Alberta Hospital to help us protect and save our teeth, for which I'm very grateful. When I was dealing with immediate frustrations like throat pain or mouth sores, the impact of radiation on my teeth was not top of mind. Now that I'm well into recovery, I'd better get on with taking care of them.

I'm thankful that my family and friends have been so supportive. I'm not surprised by the support I've received from close family, especially my sisters and brother and, of course, our kids, who have been great. However, I didn't know I had so many friends and associates who would actually care.

This experience is teaching me how compassionate some people actually are, and how "not that" I've been in my life. I'm not a bad person and I don't beat myself up for this failing but it's only now that I know what compassion looks like. Whenever one of my sisters was sick with serious illnesses such as ulcerative colitis and heart surgeries, I was never really "there" for them. Knowing my own limitations, it's not hard for me to forgive those who haven't stayed connected with me throughout this illness.

Linda has laughed and said that it's sure a good thing it was me who got sick and not her. That is so true. It's also true that this cancer experience, hard as it is, is an amazing frigging learning experience. A big one. I must've had a lot to learn. I'm learning fast, God. Learning fast. Can you let up now? This recovery's been going on for far too long.

I HAVE COME A LONG WAY
AND STILL HAVE FAR TO GO

It's been 12 days since I last wrote. Seems like a long time. Nothing dramatic. More slow, steady progress. I've kicked the morphine by reducing the amount slowly. I didn't take any yesterday or today. It's taken a few days to realize the benefits. I'm noticing that my mental energy and sense of humour are back. I can think again. It's like putting on glasses; what was blurry is clear and sharp again.

Also, I've made big strides with eating. I'm back to where I was two months ago, and maybe even better. I'm eating with far less pain and have started the countdown of the 30 days I need to go without using my feeding tube and without losing weight. Now I'm on Day Six of eating everything through my mouth. When I started the countdown, I was at 141 pounds. and am now at 142.8 pounds. My goal is to get up to 150 by Christmas. I'm eating three good meals a day and drinking two *Ensures* so that I'll get over 2,000 calories a day. I need that many to gain weight.

If someone invites us for dinner, I have to warn them that I still have trouble eating. The pain of swallowing has gone but I still find it difficult to swallow. I have to make gurgling sounds and swallow hard with every swallow. It's noisy, it's work, and it's slow-going. Plus bits and pieces of food stick in the back of my throat and I have to bring it back into my mouth with some phlegm and spit into a tissue. This goes on after the meal too. I have phlegm at the back and top of my throat most of the time so I always need a tissue nearby. Yuk! I still tend to aspirate, which makes me cough while eating. Not enjoyable for me or my dining partners. I'm getting better, but I'm not there yet.

Same with my stamina. I still tire easily but I recover much more quickly. When I was on morphine, I would take an hour to recover from an hour-long walk. Now I hardly notice I was on a walk. And I can feel my strength returning. I do a weight training program that takes me half an hour to do. I'm doing the same exercises I did before cancer, but I now use 10-pound dumbbells when it used to be 25 to 30 pounds. I started at four push-ups and am now up to eight. A long way to the 40 push-ups I used to be able to do. It may take a while, but I'm optimistic about getting my base fitness level back.

Linda and I went swimming today, and I did laps for 20 minutes, with plenty of rest in between. I'm pleased, but I know I have a lot of work to do to be ready for my surfing lessons in Costa Rica in January and February.

Our accommodations in Tamarindo are booked and I'm signed up for a week of lessons, two hours a day, so I have to be ready. Beginner lessons on beginner waves. If I can't do it, that's OK, but I feel compelled to try. My exercise program is designed for surfing fitness. I'll be strong enough, but I'm worried about my stamina. I've got to get out for rides on my fat bike and go swimming more often.

Do I still have pain? Yes, my throat still hurts on the left side where the radiation was the strongest. It's going away but not gone. Do I have the saliva problems they predicted? Yes, but not the bad dry mouth that some folks get. My saliva glands sort of work overtime so I'm getting more saliva than normal. Not a big deal, but everywhere I go, I have to bring tissues and a plastic bag along with a water bottle. I frequently have to clear my throat and spit, then wash out my mouth with a quick drink of water. Partly this is a swallowing problem, but it's also my saliva glands.

Even though I seem to have excess saliva, the saliva is thicker than normal and my teeth don't get cleaned like they did pre-radiation. So, I swish my mouth with water after every meal and make sure I brush frequently. This saliva problem may never go away. It's a pain in the ass for sure, but it could be so much worse.

What about my taste buds? I seem to be able to taste everything, but sweet is not as sweet as it used to be, pre-cancer. For a while, sugar was leaving a bad after-taste, but now it doesn't. Something more to be grateful for.

How do I look? Better than when I was on morphine but still pretty gaunt. My cheeks are hollow and I have wrinkles that I never had before. I also have jowls and a turkey neck from radiation. All head and neck patients get that; it goes away eventually. Plus the hollow cheeks will fill out when I gain weight. I look skinny, but that too will change with time. I confess to having a strange pattern of creases of loose skin all along my back. It's from drastic weight loss. Good thing I never see myself naked from behind!

Are any readers wondering about my sex drive? It went away. I missed it. But it's back. A great sign that I'm recovering. Hallelujah.

Can I drink wine or beer? No, it's just too hard on my throat. I drink water, apple juice, and that's about it. Not even coffee. I also chug an *Ensure* twice a day for the calories and protein. Not exactly a party drink.

What else? Linda's tired of looking after me. The morphine days were hard on me and hard on her too. When I came off it, I'd been used to being looked after so I seem to have just carried on being looked after. That has not gone over well. Marital tension! Good thing we're capable of getting over these difficulties. At our last support group meeting, Linda and two other wives made it clear that they're also victims of their husbands' throat cancer. They're expected to care for us, and they're OK with that, but our symptoms and needs are constantly shifting, and being a caregiver can be a drag. It's also hard to cook for us because our interest in food and our ability to eat keeps changing. Issues around food seem to be the biggest drag for the wives.

I have the CT scan coming up on Thursday. The doctor needs to confirm that the two small spots on my lungs are from food that I aspirated into my lungs and not cancer. Here's some good news. The Oilers are back on track after losing a few games. And you just spent 10 minutes reading this without having to read or think about Donald Trump. He's such an attention hog.

CANCER-FREE
AND FEELING UNSTOPPABLE

I got the CAT Scan results from my doctor. I'm cancer free. The spots on my lungs were indeed infections caused by food going down my windpipe. The larger one has shrunk to half its original size. The smaller ones are arranged in a pattern typical of infection. I hadn't been worried. The doctor had told me he didn't think it'd be cancer. But, then again, you never know. I'll still need to have another scan when we get back from Costa Rica in late February, to make sure the infections have cleared themselves up.

Meanwhile, I'm in a hurry to get the feeding tube out of my stomach. After removing the tube, there's a risk of getting a hernia if I strain that area of my stomach, so I have to avoid sports and heavy lifting for six weeks after getting it out. For me to take the surfing lessons in Costa Rica they have to remove my tube this week, so it's being done two weeks ahead of schedule. The doctors cut me some slack because I've been eating full meals for a while and they trust me. And I've gained a bit of weight. I'm up to 144.5 pounds today.

As there's very little risk of getting a hernia now, I'm going snowboarding at Marmot Basin near Jasper on Sunday and maybe Monday. Linda and I will be winter camping in the Sprinter Van. I've also signed up for a beginner surfing lesson at the big wave pool at West Edmonton Mall. Who would have thought there'd be indoor surfing in Edmonton? They open up the pool to surfing three times a week at 8:00 PM, after the swimmers have gone home. I watched a few young guys surfing there a few days ago. It looked like fun. The waves appear to be the size of the waves at a beginner beach in Costa Rica, but more predictable. I think I can do it.

I'm feeling unstoppable now. Feels good.

But I'm well aware that, while I'm cancer-free, I'm going to be feeling the effects of radiation therapy for a long time. Like the rest of my life. Now that I'm over most of the drama and trauma of radiation recovery, it seems as though whatever inconvenient symptoms I'll have to deal with going forward will be a small price to pay.

I'm thankful.

MY CURRENT NORMAL

Yesterday, at my support group meeting, Franz, a new tongue cancer patient, and his wife joined our group. They talked excitedly about a tongue cancer blog they'd been reading. It turned out to be mine. I was thrilled, of course.

I'm about five months ahead of Franz in my cancer treatment, so they're finding my documentation useful in predicting what might happen to him. Anna, my swallowing coach, has said that, even though all throat cancer experiences are different, mine is pretty common, so it's instructive for many new patients.

According to my radiation oncologist, Dr. Debenham, it takes about a year from the last radiation treatment to get to the real "new normal." I'm still six months away. Here's what my current normal looks like.

The spot in my throat that the radiation damaged the most is healing well. My doctor was very pleased when he looked at it with a scope yesterday. I can still feel some pain, but not as much as before. While my throat is still sensitive to spicy foods, that also seems to be diminishing. My feeding tube is gone. I swallow with no pain. My weight has gone up to 147 pounds. I still drink two bottles of *Ensure* or *Boost* a day to keep my calorie intake up but I'm eating three meals a day. How good is that?

Plus I'm not taking any medications. My bowel movements are regular. I sleep well, without sleeping pills. Most of my problems with mucus/phlegm have gone away. I don't have to spit into a tissue, over and over, all day long, like I used to.

My facial hair is back. The hair at the nape of my neck is also back. And it's a darker color. Stylish, I think. I hope. I almost look healthy. Skinny but healthy. Not emaciated like I used to look. My cheeks have filled out, but my turkey neck is still there. Have I mentioned that radiation to the throat results in a turkey neck. I never see it, so it doesn't bother me, but I know its there. It eventually goes away.

I'm almost as energetic as I used to be, although I don't have the stamina I used to have. That'll come. I'm thankful for all the progress.

There are still issues to deal with. For example, I can taste my food, but the tastes aren't always the same as they were, especially sweets, which still start out tasting good but then leave a bad aftertaste. So many of the things I used to love to eat are now dead to me. Ice cream, cake, cookies, even fruit. And wine.

I still have problems swallowing and that may be a permanent part of my new normal. Thanks to the damage to my throat and the lack of saliva, food will often not just slip down my throat. Some gets caught in the mucus and then seems to get hung up at the back of my throat, which means I have to force it down with a drink of water. Even then, 20 minutes after a meal, there's often gunk in my throat that just won't go away. Bits of food keep backing up into my throat from my nasal passages; I have to clear my throat and spit out food bits and phlegm. Gross.

And I have to brush my teeth frequently to make them even feel clean. That's part of what's meant by "dry mouth." I don't have enough saliva to naturally clean my mouth and teeth so I have to brush after every meal and before going to bed, just to make my mouth and my teeth feel clean. That was never an issue before radiation. Now, I do a lot of brushing and swishing to clean away the bits of food that cling to my teeth and inside my cheeks just to make them even feel clean. My teeth and oral health will always require more attention than before. There are often problems with gums and soft tissue around the teeth. To protect tooth enamel and prevent cavities, I also use fluoride trays once a day. These are the same as those your dental hygienist uses when she cleans your teeth every three months. I use them every day. If I ever need tooth extractions or have any other dental surgery, it'll have to be done in a bariatric chamber for protection. Besides treating decompression sickness, hyperbaric oxygen therapy helps to heal serious infections and wounds that won't heal as a result of radiation injury. Who knew?

I often have a bad taste in my mouth after eating so the brushing and swishing help with that problem too. I follow a meal with sugar-free *Trident* gum that gets the saliva flowing and improves the taste in my mouth. We'd originally bought some expensive xylitol gum, specifically for generating saliva, at 11 bucks a package, but *Trident* seems to work just as well.

The saliva glands at the upper part of my mouth that secrete a thicker mucus-like saliva didn't get damaged by the radiation, but the glands at the lower part of my jaw that secrete a more liquid version of saliva did. Sometimes these glands never heal. If they do heal, it could take about a year from the last radiation treatment.

The biggest problem I have with eating is aspiration – liquid and sometimes food heading down the windpipe rather than the esophagus. When it happens, I cough, hack, sputter, sometimes sneeze, and sometimes end up spitting food into a tissue. By the end of a meal, bits of food will have migrated into my nostrils, which often makes me sneeze and blow my nose to clear out the food bits and mucus. It's like I have a sinus problem or cold. It seems to occur when the meal is dry, and I follow up my chewing with a swig of water. It also happens when

I'm eating stews and soups. It's liquid that gives me a problem. Pasta meals are the least likely to bother me. The noodles slide down nice and easy.

Will this problem ever go away? It could if I'm lucky; maybe doing those swallowing exercises will help me control the problem. The doctors have told me that the sensors in my throat that would ordinarily identify and block food going the wrong way are damaged. Damaged enough that I don't know if I'm aspirating or not. Still… My experience of "dry mouth" is not as bad as others in my group. I drink a lot more water than I ever did. Both to help with swallowing and to clean out my mouth. I've taken to drinking *Perrier* because I like the fizzy sensation.

Plus there's the perennial risk of food getting into my lungs and causing infection, potentially pneumonia. People die of pneumonia. Especially old people. That would be me. I'm old and getting older.

Apart from support with dental care, Alberta Health Services also provides free counselling. Maybe I'll take them up on it. Frankly, I'm not as happy as I should be considering that I just beat cancer, sold my business, and am comfortably retired with no real financial worries. On a day-to-day basis, I'm a bit sad and out of sorts. Not so it's debilitating, but I do notice it. I think it's a retirement thing. Feeling a loss of purpose. Among my worries is the fear that I may never get back to being as strong and fit as I was before cancer. That feels like a real loss. I used to enjoy the level at which I could mountain bike and snowboard. I sure hope I can get that back.

I experienced what felt like a fitness setback recently when I finally got out to Marmot Ski Hill in Jasper, Alberta. On my first few snowboarding runs I felt shaky as expected and did not go too fast or try too much so wasn't discouraged. But as I gained confidence, I tried a few of my old tricks and did not have the strength in my legs to get any pop out of them. I also found I had to stop frequently to rest my legs and catch my breath. And I was afraid to got too fast. Discouraging. Then I caught an edge attempting an easy spin move, fell backwards and banged the back of my head against the hard snow. I had a helmet on but still, that is how snowboarders get concussions. I was Ok but lay there for a long while feeling sorry for myself, "Shit, my snowboarding days are over. Am I old now? Who am I when I am not an athlete?" Eventually I got up and rode away tentatively. To play it safe I only stayed on the hill a while longer. It took a few hours to lose that 'glass half empty' feeling. Oh well. Recovery does not happen right away. I just need more time on my board to get my grove back. I'll get lots of boarding in on the riverside ski hills in Edmonton before I go on that cat skiing trip in March.

Right now, I'm on a fitness program that involves swimming every second or third day plus some resistance training and yoga to prepare me for learning how to surf. Learning to surf has been on my bucket list for a long time. Since we're going to Costa Rica, now's the time to do it. Linda deserves to holiday near beaches and flowers, so I need to switch from snowboarding to surfing. Surfing is hard; the most demanding part is paddling out to catch the waves. I worry that I may not be fit enough for much paddling. If I become good enough to ride beginner waves, that'll satisfy me.

After we get back from Costa Rica, Linda and I are planning to go with friends to Sunshine Ski Resort near Banff so I can snowboard for a few days. I need to prepare for the cat ski/boarding trip I've planned with the young guys I went with last year. I want to be in good enough shape to snowboard with them even if I can't exactly keep up with them.

Anyway, it's good to have goals to work toward, like surfing in January and snowboarding in March. It motivates me to do my daily workouts. I did 16 good push-ups yesterday. Up from five a month ago.

One more change to add to my new normal that I've already mentioned is that my voice is lower and deeper. That wouldn't be such a big deal, but Linda often can't hear me because her hearing aids don't pick up my voice in its new range. It's frustrating for both of us and it makes communication harder. Communication has never been an issue for us. Now it is.

On another note, as a lifetime reminder that I've survived

this cancer, when they took the feeding tube out they left what looks like a belly button above my real belly button. I now have a second belly button. Weird.

SURFING COSTA RICA STYLE

We're now in Costa Rica where we'll be spending most of January and February with Linda's twin sister, Lorna, and her husband, George, who've just moved from Atlanta, Georgia to a town called Atenas near San Jose. They've bought a lovely, small house on an acreage with a beautiful view of the valley. Great as it is to see them, I'm on a mission. I'm here to surf. Linda, our trip planner, made sure to put lots of surfing spots on our agenda.

We start out in Tamarindo, surf mecca of Costa Rica. It's full of surf shops. Our hotel guy introduced us to the Costa Rica Surf Shop, run by his friends Sonjia and Diego, who have given us an instructor named Julio. Julio is a good-looking, super-fit 25-year-old from Venezuela – a really nice guy. He's a displaced oil trade worker, happy now to be teaching surfing and playing bongos in a band. His girlfriend is pregnant; they're a joyful pair.

We pay only $43, almost half what most shops charge. Julio says that includes the board rental for the day, but after a one-and-a-half-to-two-hour lesson, I won't want to go out again. He was right. Nonetheless, he's impressed that I'm almost 69 and learning to surf. His dad is 65 and fit, but will not surf. To Julio, surfing is the ultimate sport. Everyone should learn it.

He started me with dry land training. I'd seen it all before on YouTube videos that demonstrate the "pop up" technique, and had already been practicing it 15 or 20 times a day in our living room. We then began working with a board that was 10 feet long. Made of foam. Stable and best for beginners. We walked out into the water to an area near some body surfers. The waves were beginner waves. Maybe three feet high. They came in groups of four or five, with lots of flat water in between. The water was colder than I'd expected and I was glad I'd brought my "shorty" wet suit. I'm skinny, and I knew I'd be cold. Julio wore one too; we were the only ones to do so.

He showed me how to walk the board out to where the body surfers were, and how to lift the nose when the waves came in. There were a few other beginner surfers out there too, but they didn't have instructors and were struggling. We started where the water was chest high. Good, I wouldn't have to exhaust myself paddling.

He showed me how to pull myself up onto the board from the side and to position myself relative to the markers on the board – a line down the middle, a mark that my chin should be positioned above. He told me to place my hands to the side of my chest. Don't grab the board.

Feet touching each other. Toes on the board.

He read the waves and lined the board up facing the shore so he could push me with the wave. As he pushed, the wave caught the board, I felt a rush, and the front of the board started racing. It was fast. He yelled, "Get up!" I arched my back like I'd practiced, brought my feet up under me, and got up. I was up and almost balanced for a short ride and then I fell backwards. Julio was impressed. He said my front foot had to be more forward. We walked back to our start point. The next few rides were the same. Up and fall. Up and fall. Things happened so fast I wasn't sure if my front foot was coming up further or not. Finally, I got a longer ride going. I fell and he told me my back arm was behind me like a snowboarder, not with the elbow bent forward like a surfer. I said I would try but in fact there were too many little things to think about and it all happened so fast. A surfboard is much less stable than a snowboard.

Next time I got up, I felt balanced for the first time, and I felt as though I was actually surfing. Julio yelled, "Bend your legs!" I dropped down deeper and was pleased that my balance improved. I had a moment of being proud and the ride ended with me pitching to the side. Julio was excited for me like a good instructor should be, and praised me for being a fast learner. Even the body surfers noticed my long ride.

The next three tries were short. I was losing concentration

and suggested we go in for a rest. We found Linda, who enthusiastically applauded my efforts. Since we had another half hour of lessons left, we went out again.

The first ride I got up quickly and was going well when I noticed that the board was going parallel to the wave behind me – not perpendicular like Julio says a long board was supposed to be. I made a quick, automatic adjustment like I would on a snowboard. All of a sudden, the board and I were rushing toward the beach. I crouched lower and think, "I'm surfing!" It was a long run, but of course I fell. I got up and flexed my muscles in celebration toward Linda, who was on the beach.

Julio and I celebrated and congratulated each other on the way back out. He was pleased. The next rides were not so successful but still promising. Finally, I had another long ride, like a real surfer, and I made it almost all the way to the beach. I fell off where the sand was only six or eight inches below the water. Nice!

The next few times, I lost my concentration. Julio said the wind was causing us problems. We tried one more wave and it was a good enough ride to quit on. It'd been a successful lesson. Linda was impressed. Julio said I would be exhausted and would need a day of rest. He was right.

That night, over a nice dinner that Linda had prepared, I asked her if she'd seen my long rides and if I looked like a surfer. She answered with a kind smile and said, "You looked like an old man who's learning how to surf." I'll take that. During our time in Tamarindo, I surfed with Julio five more times and got a bit better at it but never really very good. I was able to ride longer but eventually realized that standing on the board was the easy part. The hard part was catching the wave. Having Julio reading the waves for me, telling me when to paddle and when to pop up, and even giving me a little push was what made me think I could surf.

I really hoped to learn how to read the waves, to time my paddling, and to pop up without Julio's help. No chance. Even after about 15 lessons with a guide, whenever I tried surfing on my own, I found I still needed to have an experienced guide saying, "This is the one, it's a good wave, go, go, go, paddle, paddle, paddle, pop up, pop up!" Left to my own devices, I'd think I had a good wave and had timed it right, only to find that it was a weak wave or too big and that I'd started paddling too late or too early. I'd just fail to get up and would have to regroup and get ready to try another wave, only to have it happen again and again. Every now and then I'd get up. It's a lot of work and frustration, especially for an old man who's been weakened by cancer.

During the next three weeks, Linda and I traveled to two or three other beaches in Costa Rica and Panama. I got out on the water with new instructors for an hour or two each time. I improved but never to the point where I could read the waves and get myself up on my own. The instructors cost me $45 and were well worth it. They loved teaching me because I was an old man who was able to get up on a wave and ride it for a while. Although they were only beginner waves, it still wasn't easy.

I loved being on the beach living the surfer dream for the moment, but frankly this was the hardest sport I'd ever tried. Snowboarding and mountain biking are way less demanding. As a mountain biking friend later told me, "Surfing is the least rewarding sport you'll ever try. And maybe the most rewarding when you finally get up."

I had fun, I'm glad I did it, and I'll do it again any time Linda wants to go to a warm sunny place with ocean beaches. If I can rent a board with an instructor who can find me good beginner waves, then I'm a surfer. Well, a beginning surfer. It's now my winter get away sport.

The next part of our trip was Panama where I took surf lessons in Playa Venao for a few days before going to visit my sister and brother-in-law in Punta Chame, where Gary goes to kite ski every winter. I guess I could take up kite skiing. Gary, who's only a couple of years younger than me, seems to love it. Maybe too much gear and too technical for me. And wind, I don't like wind. I'd rather be learning how to surf. I can play around on a rented board on beach holidays while I keep snowboarding as my primary winter sport and mountain biking as my way of staying in shape.

When we get back to Edmonton there'll still be some winter left for me to get in more snowboarding. Then there's my annual trip to Retallack near Nelson BC for cat skiing and snowboarding. It should be epic.

I DIDN'T DO THIS ALONE

It's been a challenging, eight-month-long journey from discovering I had tongue cancer to where I am today – cancer-free and almost at my "new normal." The list of people to thank is long. Check out my Acknowledgments page, if you don't believe me. Medical staff who cared for me, my cancer support group who inspired me, my devoted family who loved me unconditionally, friends who touched my heart and made me laugh, business colleagues who had my back, healers who eased my pain, snowboard and mountain biking buddies who kept up my morale, veteran tongue cancer survivors who shared their courage and wisdom, blog followers who stayed the course… It took more than a village to get me here.

What about Linda? Shouldn't I thank her? There'll never be enough words for all that I should thank her for. She took care of everything while I was recovering. She's also such wonderful company. I'm blessed to have this wise, funny, and beautiful woman in my life. I look forward to travelling with her in our retirement. We'll be that happy retired couple living like nomads.

SHOWING UP IS SHOWING OFF

I've been envisioning attending this year's annual cat ski and snowboarding trip as my victory lap after beating cancer and surviving a tough year. It's been my recovery goal for the last few months. Exactly a year ago, I came home from this same trip at Retallack, a cat ski resort near Nelson, BC, feeling elated and proud of myself, only to come crashing down when I discovered I had tongue cancer.

Of course, all 24 of the guys and the guides and staff at Retallack were full of compliments, impressed that I'd come back so soon to challenge the steep mountain runs and the deep snow. They made me feel glad I was there. There were concerns about my strength and stamina. I was convinced I could handle it. I was wrong.

The last thing Linda said on my way out the door was, "Don't try and show off to those young guys. In your case, showing up is showing off." She was right, as she always is. The best thing I did was show up. That turned out to be good enough.

After my first run through the deep snow and trees it was clear to the guide, and to me, that I had overestimated my strength and ability. It was time to recalibrate. At the top of the hill, I'd been confident. It looked steep and there were trees beneath me, but there were openings between the trees that I knew I could navigate through. The snow looked deep and soft. I'd done it before and I could do it again. Wrong. I had trouble with my toe side turns in the deep snow and soon I was picking up too much speed and had to fall as a way of stopping. Once I'd fallen, I realized that getting up would be hard. The snow was deeper, wetter, and heavier than last year. My ski buddy, Sandy, helped pull me up using his ski poles. I got up but my snowboard was embedded under the heavy snow. I struggled to get the front end up and free of the snow so I could start again. It took effort and time, but eventually I got going.

I fell three or four more times on the way to the bottom where the others were waiting. I felt a bit embarrassed at making them wait but I was ready for another run. The falls were not dramatic. Getting up was difficult each time and, yes, it drained my energy, but I felt that my riding was getting better as we approached the end of the run. I was confident I would get myself under control the next run. The first run is always the hardest.

Back in the cat, I got into a deep discussion with Joey Hundert, one of the superb skiers, about "flow experiences" and about how skiing and snowboarding can get you into a flow state. After the discussion, he decided he'd be my partner on the next run. I welcomed riding with Joey because he's a star and I guess I was also trying to impress him with my riding, or at least my courage. Silly me. How could I will myself into a flow state before I'd even established that I could snowboard in this deep wet snow? I tried to get myself into a rhythm and ride faster than I was really capable of riding. It was exhilarating when I was hitting my turns, but scary when I got out of rhythm and started losing control.

Once out of control, of course I'd fall. Joey pulled me up, and away I'd go again. I fell twice with no consequence, but the last two falls were into tree wells. Tree well falls are dangerous. Once you're in a tree well, a snow-covered deep hole around the base of a big tree, you need help to get out. The snow is deep and there's nothing to grab onto for leverage. If you fall face first, you can be in trouble. People suffocate in tree wells. Both times I fell backwards and slipped into a hole under the lower tree branches down into the deep snow. My board stayed uphill with my body and head below. My face was not buried, so I was OK, but I was disoriented. I was deep in snow, wedged under the big branches with my back against the trunk. I was also embarrassed. This is what the guides warn everyone about. Getting out was exhausting. Both times, with lots of help from Joey and the guide, Chris, I managed to get my snowboard off and to squirm up and out of the tree well. Once out, I had the challenge of strapping my boots to the board. With all that wet snow built up in my bindings I struggled to get the bindings to connect. More frustration. Deeper exhaustion.

I realized that much more of this would sap all my already limited energy. I was not as strong as I needed to be. It was taking me way too long to get down this run. There were guys waiting at the cat who'd paid big money for this adventure trip. The guilt of wasting their valuable cat skiing time weighed as heavily on me as the deep wet snow. I watched Joey ski through the trees like he was in a beer commercial and it made me very conscious that I was riding with some elite skiers and riders, and I was holding them up.

At the bottom, I talked to Chris and Savage, our guides, and we decided I'd wait out the next few runs. The idea was to find runs that were more open, with fewer trees, and maybe flatter so the boarding would be less challenging. That never happened. The avalanche danger was high that day so the wide-open areas were too dangerous. We could only ski safely in the steeper, tree-protected runs. So, I stayed in the cat. One of the other skiers, Sean, had issues with his equipment, so he sat out the rest of the day with me. At least I had company.

The next day I drove to a local ski hill, two hours away, with Tommy Kalita. Tommy comes on the trip for the social life and networking, but doesn't feel comfortable cat skiing so he drives to Whitewater, a regular ski hill near Nelson. We had fun. I can ride the groomed runs all day long and enjoy it. It's the steep and the deep I can't handle. Yet. When we got off the groomed trails and into the tree areas, the snow was hard and no fun to ride so we avoided the trees. We drove back to Retallack feeling good about our day. We arrived just as the two cats were getting back to the lodge. When I saw how happy the guys were getting out of the cats, I was jealous. Everyone had had a great time, including the guys I was sure I could keep up with. I wanted some of that.

I decided right then that I was going with them the next day and I told the guides. The guides accepted my decision, probably with reluctance. Next morning, the head guide assured me it was OK with them, but as we talked, I could tell he had concerns. The avalanche danger was worse today, and I realized that if there were an incident on the mountain, I might be the weak link. The guy keeping our guides from taking care of other guys.

Later, Antoine Palmer, my good friend and the organizer of the trip, sought me out, looked me in the eye, and asked if I really wanted to do this. He confirmed that Linda had been right – "showing up was showing off." No one would think less of me for not going. I already knew that, but I also had my own expectations of myself to live up to. We both knew what the wise choice was. Later, we learned that two weeks earlier, a skier at Retallack had almost suffocated in a tree well. That explained why the guides were hyper-nervous.

I went back to the Whitewater ski hill again with Tommy. We had a great time. The snow was great. I got closer to a flow experience than I would have in the steep and deep. I even got in some good tree runs. The guys in the cats also had a good time. I was envious of the other guys again but, all in all, I was OK with my ski experience. Despite not having done much cat boarding, I had a great time and got my money's worth out of the whole adventure.

The guys who do cat skiing or snowboarding tend to be interesting characters. This group of guys are all friends and associates of Antoine and Joey, so they're all amazing guys. They're living proof of the axiom, "We all become a composite of the six people we associate with the most." These guys have a lot in common. Entrepreneurial – most of them own their own companies. Successful – they're all playing at the top of their game. Caring – they treat people well. Socially conscious – they're all working toward a better world. Family-oriented or community-minded – many are married with young kids. Young – everyone is between 30 and 40 years old with one or two near 50. Fit and athletic – of course. Courageous guys who take calculated risks – guys who cat ski, own their own companies, and would still go to Burning Man.

Hanging out for five days with 24 high-performers was a treat. Over the weekend, I either took part in or overheard conversations about altered consciousness techniques for performance enhancement; the metrics used to manage an internet sales company; using toy robots to teach children about complex decision-making; the pros and cons of standard building construction processes (design build versus cost-plus build); the math of investing in commercial real estate; the appeal of open marriage and polyamorous relationships in today's crazy world; the challenges involved in designing robots that do day-to-day work; the costs and paybacks for various forms of electrical power generation; the challenges of hiring a general manager to replace yourself at work; the best places to surf; what it feels like to own a company that's about to experience exponential growth; the challenges of raising kids in junior high; the social value of hedge funds; mountain biking versus running as a fitness activity; the appeal of living in a Sprinter van; the experience of leaving a safe job to start a new company; the excitement of conceiving a product and bringing it to market; the joys and vagaries of being a dad.

Yah, we also talked about Donald Trump. (How could we ignore him?) But you get the idea. It was great fun hanging out with a bunch of young guys who live their lives on what most of us would think of as "the edge." The whole experience was inspiring. For a weekend, I felt like I was a high performer too. Being with these guys way back when my cancer was discovered, and then beating cancer, recovering from radiation, and getting back to join them in Retallack a year later was an accomplishment.

REAL LIFE IS MESSY

Nope. It's not over. I can't quit yet. This cancer experience is ongoing. It doesn't have a dramatic ending. It didn't end with my going on my cat ski trip and celebrating my victory. It would have been so perfect, wrapping up the story with a successful cat ski trip to bookend my one-year cancer journey that had begun right after the same trip a year ago. But real life is messy. It doesn't work like it does in the movies.

I sold my business, PlayWorks, and I'm happy I did, but it's a complicated sale and I still have work to do before I get all of our proceeds from the sale. A chunk of the money is tied up in the receivables for two big projects we need to collect final payments on. And Jill, the new owner, has asked the staff to plan a "retirement/beat cancer" party for me in early May. I need to give them my invitation list. It's no small matter searching names and compiling a list, complete with emails, of all the people I'd want to see there – family, friends, staff, business associates, industry people, suppliers, contractors, even competitors. And then there are my favourite former playground committee customers, landscape architects, and a whack of parks department employees. I've been running this business for over 35 years. That's a long time and a lot of people.

Linda and I are also elbow-deep in retirement planning, getting our finances in order, making travel plans, figuring out where to live, considering volunteer work, mapping out our future. We feel like twenty-somethings again. Trying to figure out what to do with the rest of our lives. We're also selling the rental duplex we own. These are problems we feel blessed to have, but they add to that feeling of, "Hey, shouldn't I have time on my hands? I'm supposed to be retired!"

But I'm a busy guy, the Oilers are on a roll, Donald Trump is talking about dropping bombs, and there are so many shows to watch on TV. I don't have time for cancer recovery. However, the recovery is not over. I've had three appointments with the health care community in the last couple of weeks that have made that point clear. The first was a trip to my dentist's office that unnerved me. I went in for my regular cleaning. I feel like I've been brushing frequently and carefully, but I found out I've not been doing enough. After the cleaning, my dental hygienist said she's already seeing signs of the enamel breaking down. This is not good. She asked if I was using my fluoride trays. First, I said "yes," but then had to admit that I'd only started to use them recently. They used to aggravate my mouth sores, but they're not bothering me anymore. I'm supposed to fill these trays, like a hockey player's mouth guards, with fluoride and put them in my mouth for five minutes. I had to admit that I'd missed a lot of nights because I'm just not in the habit of doing it. I don't make new habits easily, especially good ones. Ask Linda.

We then discussed what could happen in the long run, which made me fear the prospect of major tooth decay and losing my teeth. I intend to live another 30 years, which means I could outlive my teeth. She also showed me how to use an electric toothbrush properly. Linda bought one for me recently because it works so much more effectively than a regular toothbrush. I didn't like using it, so I didn't. You can bet I do now. I also do my fluoride treatment every night, and every night I wonder how much damage I've already done to my teeth by not having done this regularly since I started the radiation treatments.

The second meeting was with a speech therapist at the hospital where I'd gone for follow-up testing on my speech and my swallowing. I learned a lot about what my new normal will be like. Some parts of it will be hard to swallow. (Pun intended.) Just like with the fluoride trays, I'll always wonder if my swallowing would have been better if I'd done my swallowing exercises regularly. Again, I can blame it on the mouth pain, but mostly I could have done them and really should have.

The next meeting was with a psychologist. She gave me some insight into something that should have been obvious. I may be over the physical part of cancer recovery, but the psychological recovery can take much longer. It may be even harder to deal with. Now it makes sense that I'm not feeling happy, even though my cancer recovery is well along. I'm glad I asked for help.

I'd been thinking I was almost over this thing, but I should have known better. The drama of cancer discovery, radiation and chemo treatments is over, but the aftereffects keep going on and on and on.

Cancer is a major life event. So is retirement. So is selling a business. One major life event is hard enough to deal with. Linda and I are coping with three. I need to cut us some slack.

MY WORLD HAS GONE FLAT

There's something missing in my life. Everything feels flat. No fizz. I can't explain it and I don't know why I feel this way. It makes no sense. My counsellor from the Cross Cancer Institute told me that this is what depression is. Unexplainable feelings you can't get over. A sense of loss. She suggested that I was experiencing low-grade depression.

I started by telling her about where I was with cancer recovery. As I outlined it for her, it occurred to me, as it often does, that I have a good life. There's no good reason for me to be seeing a psychologist. I told her I felt guilty taking up her valuable time when she could be seeing someone in greater need. (Her services are free to cancer patients.) She said that her cancer patients often tell her that. "Don't worry," she said, "you're the type of patient we're here for."

She explained that when she came here to work with cancer patients, she was prepared to deal with trauma patients suffering through operations, radiation, chemo, and full-on drama. What she has found instead is that most of her patients are people like me – over the physical illness but dealing with low-grade depression. She said that cancer recovery is rarely the big "triumph of the human spirit" story that people expect. The arc of psychological recovery is longer than the physical recovery, and it's not dramatic.

The feelings I have aren't dramatic either; it's more of a lack of feeling, and it's pervasive. No one would notice except Linda. I don't mope. I get around and do all the normal things and look like a success. Looking good is still important, so I keep up with appearances. But there is something missing. My world is flat. Well, not completely flat but definitely flatter. I'm not as interested as I used to be. I've lost some of my lust for life. Let's deal with the "lust" part first. It's not something we dwell on, but both Linda and I know that I don't have my usual sex drive. I have the physical energy, but I've lost some of my "interest." That's a huge loss. No wonder I'm depressed. Will I get it back? I'm sure I will. If I don't, we'll adjust, but...

My psychologist used the word "anhedonia" to describe what I feel or don't feel. The opposite of hedonism. If hedonism is seeking pleasure and the full-on embracing of life, then anhedonia is its opposite. Anhedonia is the inability to experience pleasure from activities usually considered enjoyable – e.g, exercise, hobbies, singing, sex, and/or social interactions. Seems like a good word for what I'm not feeling, what I've called flatness.

The flatness is pervasive. I can sense it in almost every-thing. When I go snowboarding, I'm not as driven. I don't get out to the ski hill early in the morning; I get out there late and I quit early. I'm not as interested in improving, I don't push myself as hard, and I'm not having as much fun. I buy new books and only read the first chapter. I know that's common for lots of people, but for me it's worse than it used to be. I'm interested at first, but my interest wains and I quit reading. Then I buy another book and the same thing happens.

I used to be a hound for finding new music and adding songs to my *iTunes* playlists. Now, not so much. I hear new songs I like. I add them to my *iTunes*, but then I rarely go back and listen to them again. Every year, for the last 15 years, I've burned 20 of my favourite new songs on CDs and have given them to friends and relatives. Like inflicting my bad taste on them. This year I'm not doing it. No interest. No new songs to reveal.

When I'm out riding my mountain bike, I wonder when the magic will kick in again. Riding is more like work than the teenager fun it used to be.

I don't drink alcohol any more, and I don't miss it. To be honest, drinking was a source of hedonistic pleasure indulged in daily. Now it's gone. Hmmm… Maybe that's the problem. Not enough beer.

Do I find this loss of joy in life debilitating? No. It's just that I don't seem to care as much. I'm not present. There's no "me" there. I feel dull. I know it bothers Linda. Some people would say I've always been absent-minded, but it's more than being absentminded. It's being absent.

Now, when I miss the thread of a conversation I'm having with two or three people, I don't take the trouble to make sure I understand so I can participate fully. I let the others carry on, knowing that the conversation will go on without me. Being missing in action is bad enough in social situations, but in business meetings it's a real liability. When Linda and I are dealing with financial planners or our accountant, I find that I'm letting the conversation be carried by the other participants. Even when there's money on the line and I know I really should care, I don't. It's irresponsible behaviour.

So how do I get my joie de vivre back? My psychologist says that the trick is "not to give in to giving in." Try to "fake it 'til I make it." I guess I have to be patient with myself. Let the healing happen in its own time. I'd expected to be back to normal by now. I think everyone sort of expects me to be normal now that I've recovered, but those expectations are unrealistic. According to my psychologist, my current state is normal. Everyone thinks they'll get back to where they used to be in a year, which is naive. Recovery doesn't happen on a schedule, and besides, the expectation that I'll return to who I was before the cancer is equally naive.

If I think of depression as coming from a sense of loss, then my low-grade depression is explainable. I can't put my finger on what I've lost exactly, except that I miss the me I used to be. Maybe it's as simple as that. I'm not as engaged as I used to be, so I'm not as engaging. I want the engaging part of me back. My counsellor also pointed out the obvious. I've been through a lot of stress in the last year. I can say I conquered cancer, and I did. I can say I sold my business, and I should be proud of that. I can say I have every reason to look forward to a successful retirement. This is all true, thank God. But... parts of me are reacting to some other truths. I lost my health. I lost my business. I didn't really want to retire. I'm feeling diminished by it all, not energized. I also feel that I've lost something in my relationship with Linda. Fortunately, she is wise and knows we'll get back on track. But then again, she's been patient with me for a long time and her patience is wearing thin.

This visit to the psychologist came about because of a family fight that didn't seem to involve me. Linda and Mike had a huge blow-up two weeks ago. It brought out the worst in both of them. The yelling was more intense than anything the three of us had experienced since the kids were teenagers. It had obviously been simmering for a while.

Linda decided she'd get help and I agreed to do the same. Her counselling session revealed that her anger was toward me. I think it's justified. I've recovered physically but I haven't adjusted to the new normal. I'm not carrying my weight around here. She's still the caregiver. She needs a wife like the one I've got, but she doesn't have one. And I'm not a helpful guy around the house at the best of times. She's better at everything than I am, so she carries the load – cooking, shopping, banking, travel planning, tech work, household management, everything. I'm a passenger, if I'm being kind; a freeloader, if I'm not.

When my son Mike asked me what I do around the house, I had to answer, "Not much." Then I smiled and said, "I'm a blogger. I look after my blog. That's what I do around here." Kind of funny, but not really.

My listlessness may be a retirement issue. Us being together every day, all day long. Common retirement issues, yes, but compounded by Linda having become my caregiver before I retired. Without question, our relationship has been changed by the cancer experience. Not for the better. I used to add value around here by being fun to be with, but I've lost some of my charm.

I suspect a lot of this started when I couldn't talk. For three or four months, I had to communicate by writing everything down. I got used to the silence. Also, I lost some of my comic timing, so I quit trying to amuse her. We didn't have as much fun together during that quiet period. Of course, I was sick then. That's no fun either. Since my voice came back, we've picked it up and we have more fun, but I would say that the fun level is less than it was before I got sick. There's also Linda's hearing. Even when she's wearing her hearing aids, making sure she hears me is work for me, and making sure she understands what I'm saying is work for her. Sometimes we don't make the effort.

Linda is experiencing major life events just like I am. Taking care of me as a cancer patient is only one of them. Selling a business was a huge stressor. She was fully engaged in that. Facing retirement has been huge for her too. We're also getting old. I'm having trouble adjusting to that fact of life. Illness, selling my business and retirement have compounded that concern for me. On a bad day, I can feel myself drifting into old age and irrelevance. It's not surprising that Linda and I have challenges. Good thing we're still optimistic. Good thing we've both established good life habits that will carry us forward. Neither of us is inclined to let things fester; we take action. After I saw the psychologist, I felt better. Knowing that anhedonia is normal for cancer patients is comforting. It's a recovery stage that I didn't anticipate, but I will recover from it too.

Writing about all of this has been therapeutic. When I get into the flow of writing, I feel joy. Who knew there'd be hedonism in writing? Bring it on.

THINGS ARE PICKING UP

I got a lot of support after blogging about my low-grade depression. Those who'd experienced cancer in their lives didn't seem surprised. My sons were the among the first to respond. Both asked if I wanted to talk. I appreciated that. One of the most empathetic comments was from Bryan, one of the F'n riders. He appreciated my sharing as much as I had about my personal life and family struggles and assured me that other families, including his, go through the same stuff. He got me thinking about why I'm telling my story, and why I'm willing to write honestly and openly about my experiences. A lot of people find that hard and they've told me that I'm very brave, but it's not a stretch for me. It's just what I'm like. I've always wanted to be liked and I've always believed that if people understood me they would like me. That hasn't always been the case, but it's what I still believe.

When I first met and fell in love with Linda, she was surprised by how much like her girlfriends I was. I told her that's because I'm part girl. I have the female penchant for talking about feelings. I do what most men won't;

I disclose who I am. I'm comfortable divulging a lot of information about myself in exchange for something from the other person. I trust that most people will reciprocate and be kind, so I don't feel like I'm taking a big risk. I've found that being open invites others to be open with me. I'm not stupid about it though. I don't disclose everything. Just enough to be understood, to be interesting, and to get at the truth of what's going on. It's a good way of sorting out who I want to hang out with. I like people who like the real me.

The hard part for me is not the disclosure itself, but the actual writing it down so that my readers understand what I'm going through and find it interesting. I'm trusting that if you've read this far, I've succeeded.

As for my overall recovery, I'm feeling better. As soon as I wrote the last blog, things picked up. Linda and I talked. I'm now committed to contributing more to household management and tasks. Obviously, that has to happen, and it will. Also, Linda and I are now seeing my counsellor together. When you are going through a life-altering event, it's good, if not essential, to get professional counselling. How great that our medical system provides counselling for cancer patients! Who knew?

Things seem better. Blogging about my anhedonia got me lots of attention. Attention always perks a guy up. All me, all the time! Maybe it isn't healthy, but it feels good. The drama's been over for a while and I've survived. Many would have said it should be easy street from here on in, including me!

Not! Healing is not simple. There's still my low-grade depression to deal with. Boring. And the other part of my recovery, the physical part, is proving to be more of a challenge than I'd anticipated. Also, boring. My swallowing problems aren't going away any time soon. Maybe never. So now, it's about learning how to live with them and minimizing the risks associated with aspiration. I've been through a bunch of swallowing tests and am now working on exercises to improve my swallowing. More on that later.

Some of Linda's and my time has been spent helping PlayWorks plan my retirement and beat cancer celebration, less than a month from now. Something to look forward to.

HAVE I BEAT CANCER?

Everywhere I go these days, I run into people who know about my cancer. They tell me how good I look and ask how I'm feeling. Since I look and feel good, it seems to them that I've beat this thing. They're only partly right. I've won the big battle, if that's what it is, but in some important ways the fight continues. The issues I'm dealing with are subtle and hard to explain in social settings. I just end up saying I still have swallowing issues.

But from a medical standpoint I've beat cancer. I'm cancer free, it will never come back, and my recovery from radiation is almost complete. Yes, I have radiation damage that I won't recover from and there are some long-term implications, but I've essentially beat this thing.

Most of the time, I feel great. My mood has shifted; I don't seem to have that low-grade depression any more. The counselling helped. Talking it through with Linda helped. Blogging about it helped. Maybe the Oilers winning some hockey games helped. It also helped to get out on my bike and get riding.

I'm pretty healthy now. I'm eating three big meals a day. My swallowing troubles limit some foods I can eat, but I eat well. Linda is now cooking us meals to help her lose weight. Low-calorie meals. So I supplement those meals with my own food to get up to my 3,500 calories a day for weight gain. Bonus! I get to eat a lot of high calorie foods without worrying. I don't need to say no to foods like cheese, ice cream, cashews, and butter that I used to have to set limits on. I need the calories, I need the protein, so I just say yes! My weight is up to 150 pounds at 16% body fat now. I could add a few pounds of muscle and I continue to work on that.

I still do high intensity interval training workouts, 14 minutes a day. One day upper body and the next day lower body. All are body weight exercises except for a few I do with dumbbells. Go hard for a minute, rest for half a minute, and go hard again – for a total of 14 minutes. Going hard means going to 85% of capacity, but I just go 'til I'm out of breath. The regime is working; I'm getting stronger. I can do 36 push-ups and two full pull-ups – incredible progress from six months ago when I could only do four push-ups and no pull-ups.

A week ago, the single-track mountain bike trails in Edmonton's river valley dried up and I could get out on my bike again. I've been out riding four times in the last week and have ridden stronger each time. On a whim, I joined a Hardcore Bikes Club Monday night ride to see if I could cut it. I surprised myself and rode for two hours.

Sure, I was with the slow group but three of the 12 riders we started with dropped out. I didn't. And I climbed a couple of the steep hills that have always challenged me.

I've been out with other riders three times since then and I've almost held my own. I'm lighter so it's easier to climb those steep hills than it used to be. But I'm not kidding myself. It'll be hard to get my base fitness levels up to where I can ride hard with my friends in the F'n riders. It'll take time on the wheels. Maybe a year. Raising my base fitness level up to theirs is going to take a lot of work. Work I'm prepared to do.

Spring is here! The ice is off the river. Linda and I'll be out kayaking again soon. We'll also be touring in our Sprinter van. Life is good.

IT'S NOT ALL GOOD

My new normal has complications. Two issues – my swallowing and my teeth. Both are a consequence of radiation, both are long-term, and both will always be with me. There are things I can do to minimize their impact – it means adopting some new good habits. Thankfully there's no quit in me.

First the teeth issues. There are two. Radiation to the throat area has weakened the bones that the teeth are embedded in. I'm not experiencing any loss now, but I've been assured that I will. The dental people don't talk about "if" I lose my teeth; they talk about "when." When I need extractions, they'll be done in a special bariatric chamber to prevent infection. When I was first diagnosed, the dental department at the hospital took extensive pictures of my face, jaw and teeth and they've recently taken another set. They'll need them for their records in order to track the changes that will occur over time.

My friend Freda, who had throat cancer twelve years ago, just emailed to say that some of her teeth are breaking. She's also having difficulty getting used to her lower dentures, but there's no quit in that lady. Despite her teeth problems, she still seems cheerful and active at 77 years of age. She hopes the treatments are more effective these days and that I won't have the teeth problems she's experiencing. Unlike me, Freda was never offered fluoride trays, which I use every day. She was never warned about dental issues.

My friend Gary, in Vancouver, who also had radiation for tongue cancer, mentioned in an email that he'd broken a tooth recently. I guess that's likely to happen to me too. My teeth are much more prone to decay and cavities. Radiation damage to my saliva glands means that saliva isn't cleaning my teeth like it used to. It's called dry mouth, but it doesn't mean that my mouth is dry all the time. I do have saliva, but not as much as I need. To generate more saliva, I chew gum almost all the time. I'm not sure chewing gum is so great for my digestive system, but it sure seems to help with saliva. The gum also keeps my mouth fresh. Another gift from dry mouth is bad breath; thankfully, no one's complained yet.

I also have a tedious, time-consuming teeth-cleaning routine I have to follow. Every morning and every evening, I have to clean between my teeth with a pick, brush for at least two minutes with an electric toothbrush, and then floss. Every evening I also do a four-minute fluoride treatment, and then I have to wait for half an hour after that before I can eat or drink. I'm supposed to rinse my mouth with a fluoride mouthwash after eating, but I always forget. I used to be a "brush twice a day and floss now and then" kind of guy, but I'm now on a serious dental care regime. A month ago, my dental hygienist cleaned my teeth and announced that I already have decay showing. That kind of scared me into following my new regime. Fear works.

Now for the second big issue – my swallowing problems. Like all the stuff happening in our bodies, swallowing is more complicated that we realize. I used to just gulp my food down and not think about it. I still eat too fast and forget to concentrate on swallowing. When I do that, I pay a price. If the food is a thick and heavy like bread or potatoes, the price could be my throat getting so clogged up I choke, which is unnerving, to say the least. When that happens, I tell myself to stay calm and then I relieve the congestion with my ever-present glass of water. If my ever-present glass of water is absent, it's scary.

This shit happens because my natural swallowing mechanisms have been damaged by the radiation. The nerves in my throat aren't sensing what's going on like they used to. Because my nerves and muscles don't communicate effectively, the food just doesn't get pushed down as readily. It can get stuck at the top of my throat. Unless I think about each swallow, I can't tell if the food is going down. It just sits at the top of my throat and can get caught there for a long time before a swallow ends. Often I can't tell if the swallow has actually happened. Even after a meal is over, there can be food particles and gunk in my mouth, throat and nose, which can require 10 minutes of throat clearing, nose blowing, water swishing, and spitting to eliminate. It's particularly disgusting when food particles find their way into my nasal passages. Then my nose gets runny like I've got a bad cold. I blow my nose with that ever-present tissue, which gets full of snot and bits of food. Gross stuff, I know. I also do a lot of spitting into the sink. Same issue. Sometimes the food particles in my nasal passages make me sneeze, like a tickle in your nose will do. If I have a mouth full of food, that can be messy and embarrassing. It doesn't happen often any more. I'm smart enough to catch it.

If I'm having clear broth, or even juicy fruit like oranges or pineapples, the liquid can slip into my windpipe during my swallow, which will cause me to cough. It used to happen a lot, but I'm more careful now. Also, I have a new swallowing technique to keep it from happening. About a month ago, I had my six-month check-up and did a bunch of swallowing tests at the Misericordia hospital. The speech therapist, Georgina, had me swallow liquids of a variety of consistencies and captured images of my swallow on what looked like an ultrasound. We watched the images together, and she interpreted them. What I learned wasn't good. In her expert opinion, I was aspirating more than we'd previously thought. What's causing the liquid to go down the windpipe? The answer is that my epiglottis, the cartilage that covers the windpipe as food or liquids go past, has become fibrous from the radiation. This means it has hardened and can't completely fold over the entrance to my windpipe. Hence the liquid can slip down. What happens then? I cough. Usually a sudden, involuntary, hard cough. This drives the liquid back up and out. According to Georgina, sometimes the involuntary cough doesn't happen, I don't know that I'm aspirating, and the liquid goes down to my lungs. The nerves in my throat have also been compromised by radiation so they're not as sensitive as they used to be. What are the consequences? Since the liquids coming from my mouth are full of bacteria, there's always a risk of inflammation or infection in my lungs. I have more bacteria than usual because the saliva not only doesn't clean my teeth, it doesn't clean my mouth either.

As I've said, lung infections can lead to pneumonia. Once you get pneumonia a few times, you become susceptible to getting it more easily. Over the long haul, pneumonia can kill you. Do I have to worry about dying of pneumonia any time soon? No, but I do have to guard against getting it and to be hyperalert about avoiding inflammation or infection in my lungs. Georgina says that the best protection against pneumonia is healthy lungs. Note to self: Never quit mountain biking.

Georgina also expressed concern that liquids getting into my lungs would cause some of the cells to die, which would cause a gradual hardening in my lungs. That can't be a good thing. She painted a bit of a nightmare scenario for me. If I'm aspirating too much or too often, I could end up eating all of my meals through a feeding tube. Am I at that point? No, but I could tell she was worried. She said if I were ever hospitalized and for some reason was unable to sit up straight, I would need to be fed through a tube to my stomach. I got the impression that this could be a serious problem someday.

What can I do about it? Swallowing exercises. Georgina sent the results to Anna, my swallowing coach, with instructions to get me back to doing daily exercises to strengthen my swallow muscles and to change how I swallow. It will take time and effort, and it may not work but it's well worth the try. Anna seems more confident than Georgina that I can overcome this. Anna has a graduate student, Anita, who now works with me once a week. Anita seems confident too.

One of the key things that Anna and Anita do is hook me up to an instrument that graphs the quality of my swallow. The graph shows the breathing sequence and the strength of each swallow. I do an exercise and then I look at the graph to see if I did it right. That way I'm getting the feedback on my swallow that I'm not getting from my senses. Doing this repeatedly, I'm learning to hold my breath as I swallow and I'm getting a sense of what swallowing feels like so I can adapt.

I now have breathing sequence exercises and two muscle-strengthening exercises, one for my tongue and another for my throat muscles. I do 30 repetitions of these every day, which takes a full half hour. Not too long, but it's hard to get into the habit of doing them. Linda will tell you I don't create good habits easily.

Here are the three exercises. The first one is complicated. The other two are easy.

1. Take a sip of water and hold it in my mouth. Then, take in some air and hold it. Before I take in another breath, I must swallow hard, swallow again, and then clear my throat and clear it again. If the swallow doesn't feel complete, then I have to cough hard.

The idea is to hold my breath until the swallowing is done and my throat is cleared so that no liquid gets down the windpipe.

In this exercise, I'm engaging or closing off the vocal folds in my voice box to stop any liquid that has gotten past my epiglottis from getting into my lungs. The purpose of clearing my throat is to move the liquid back up and out of the windpipe. If there's still liquid in my air passage, the hard cough will drive it out. If I cough involuntarily or if I feel a tickle in my throat, the cause is the liquid being where it's not supposed to be.

I'm supposed to repeat this sequence 30 times without coughing or feeling that tickle. So far, I cough as often as six times in 30, and as few as three. I'm getting better.

2. Swallow hard 30 times while biting the front of my tongue. This is to strengthen the tongue and to help the tongue and back of my throat squeeze together tightly when I swallow.

3. Blow into a little hand-held gizmo that strengthens my throat muscles. It provides resistance, so I need to blow hard in order to get air to go through it. I stop when the air flows. When I can do it easily, we adjust the gizmo so it's hard to do again. I blow into it 30 times each session. Over time, I will gradually adjust the gizmo so the resistance gets harder and harder and my throat muscles get stronger and stronger. Anita says there's good evidence that this works to improve my swallowing.

Like everything that's good for you, any diet or exercise program, these exercises are easy to do, but even easier to not do. The consequences for failing to do the work are not immediate, so I have to create a daily routine around doing them. I have to be disciplined. Does everyone with tongue cancer, or radiation to the throat area experience these same swallowing problems. No. Some do, most don't. I do.

Others have different problems. Like not being able to speak. Georgina tested me extensively for these issues with my voice. I'm all good. No problem talking. That's a blessing. Another potential problem is malfunctioning taste buds. Luckily, mine work well. In fact, they've changed for the better and I'm enjoying food more than

I used to. An unexpected blessing. Sure, I have saliva issues, but they could be so much worse. Other patients have dry mouth that's much harder to live with than mine. I have much to be thankful for.

CELEBRATING!

Linda and I have summer trips planned in our Sprinter van which we now call "The Casita" (Spanish for little house). We're spending June on Vancouver Island and in Vancouver for a wedding, then we're meandering back to Edmonton. After the Edmonton Folk Festival, we head east, visiting folks along the way, spending time in Toronto and Montreal, then going to the Maritimes. It will be a cross-Canada tour but we plan to come home via the US after visiting friends in Maine and Boston. We'll be home in late October, I suspect. Linda and I are really looking forward to travelling. We're glad I'm feeling up for new adventures.

Plus we had one heck of a party to celebrate my retirement and beating cancer. I'm grateful to Jill White, the new owner of PlayWorks, for suggesting and hosting it. It was a goodbye to my business life and to the hard part of my recovery. About 100 people showed up to celebrate. My family, PlayWorks employees, former customers, landscape architects, F'n riders, Pow-Pow Crushers, some of my caregivers from the Cross Cancer Institute, and a wide range of Linda's and my friends from various parts of our lives. It was nice to visit with so many new friends and to reconnect with old friends from the past. In the pictures, everyone seems to be having fun and I'm grinning and laughing in every photo. I remember feeling deliriously happy.

It wasn't all drinking, music and dancing. There were speeches too. I ambushed my son, Jeff, into taking on the master of ceremonies role without giving him a sense of what the schedule would be. I told him, "We'll just make it up." I owe him big. I was praised by former colleagues in the playground industry, I was gifted with a $1000 Air Canada gift certificate by Jill, and I was flattered by Pow-Pow Crusher guys who oversold my less than heroic snowboarding moments. I was taken to task by my mountain biking buddies for stiffing them with the beer tab after my first ride with them 14 years ago. I was humbled by a loyal business friend who helped me get PlayWorks out of the ditch at its lowest moment, and I was lied about by my sister Shenta, who insisted I could walk up a flight of stairs on my hands when I was in my teens. I couldn't, but she insisted I could. Oh well. Helps build my legend. Plus, I was laughed at – a lot. Or were they laughing with me?

Linda got the biggest laugh when she insisted that this was the last get-together she was organizing for me. She said she wasn't even going to organize my funeral.

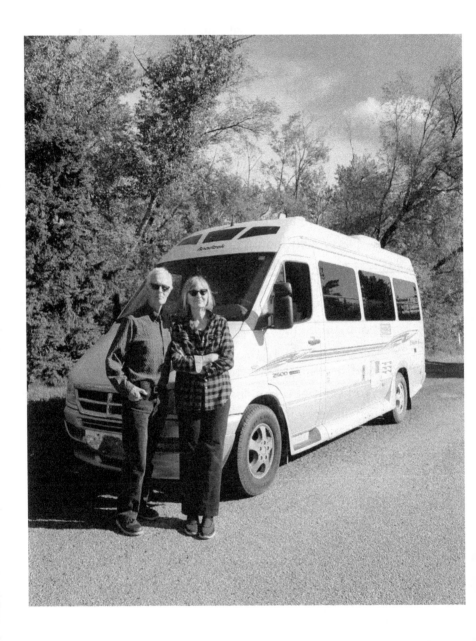

LESSONS LEARNED: NORMAL IS NOT WHAT IT USED TO BE

- You probably have more supporters than you would ever allow yourself to believe.

- Use your dreams of a better future to motivate your self to do the difficult things you need to do today.

- There is always the possibility for "joy" on the other side of recovery.

- Real life is messy. Scenarios do not unfold with cut and dried endings like in the movies.

- The arc of physical recovery from a major illness is often shorter than the arc of psychological recovery.

- If you go through a major illness you will lose some thing that has to be grieved.

- Exercise speeds both physical and psychological recovery.

- Social engagement speeds both physical and psychological recovery.

- Major illness will change you in ways that make you better as well as worse.

- Invite your supporters to celebrate your recovery and your journey.

- Life goes on.

LINDA'S CAREGIVER NOTES:

I was getting frustrated dealing with the constantly changing needs that John was presenting to me. I was anxious for him to be better and less reliant on me. After more than six months of caregiving, I was spent.

Providing nutritious food was something I could do to contribute to John's recovery, so it felt like a personal rejection when John wouldn't or couldn't eat the meals I had prepared. His tastes in food kept changing.

Several of the wives in the support group experienced this as well. As we watched our spouses struggle with their recovery, we just wanted to help but it wasn't always possible.

It isn't just the physical caregiving that is a challenge. There is a lot of emotional caregiving and that can be very draining. I continue to worry that John is not following the prescribed regimes for his teeth or that he could potentially choke while eating. I dread the day that I may have to perform the Heimlich maneuver on him.

Grieving the loss of a former life happens for both the patient and the caregiver. This is not how I thought either of us would be spending our early retirement days. Our relationship had changed, and we had to build a new way of being together as a couple. John's retirement contributed to the challenges because, at work, he had employees to do things for him and now he only had one "employee" – ME!

My world had been turned upside down and it was depressing. I found it hard to adjust to our "new normal." I should have reached out for help sooner but seeking help is not something I do easily.

A caregiver also needs care from time to time. We eventually met with a counsellor – first individually and then together. This helped us understand what we were grappling with and it opened up our communication.

The cancer changed our roles, which impacted our romantic relationship. The changes in John's mouth affected how I felt about kissing him. We had always had a good romantic relationship but now I was John's caregiver, not his lover. Our feelings about each other had changed and we had to find a way to recover the romance. Talking helps and that's what we have always been good at.

Sometimes, I felt guilty about not doing enough, especially when people would talk about how much I did for John. John felt guilty for expecting so much of me. Eventually I realized that I was doing more than I needed to be doing, and John had to learn to look after himself again. It is all a delicate balance, but we have the rest of our lives to get it right.

MOVING ON

In late May, Linda and I started the first leg of our retirement travel plan by driving our Casita to Vancouver Island. This trip was supposed to last a month, but we had such a great time on Vancouver Island, we decided to stay. We bought a condo in Comox, BC. Now we live here.

We've really enjoyed furnishing our new home, with its stunning, unobstructed view of water, trees and mountains. The Comox valley is a great retirement area for those who enjoy outdoor activities. Ocean, mountains, trees, rivers, great weather, no winter. What's not to like?

I'm mountain biking a lot. I've found some new guys to ride with here. They're not as competitive as the F'n riders, but I don't need the competition, just the camaraderie. And I've been snowboarding almost every second day since mid-December. My snowboarding companions are killing it in the deep snow, but I'm not. I still don't have the skills to ride deep powder. Maybe I never will. Maybe it's an age thing. I turned 70 while snowboarding with a friend on a ski hill called Mount Cain, riding in knee deep powder that I couldn't handle. Humbling. Still I was proud to be out there.

In September, my 96-year-old mother had a brain bleed and wasn't going to recover, so she requested and was granted an assisted death. She was a vibrant woman who had no quit in her either, but she wasn't stupid about it. She was dizzy, in pain, and had no hope of recovery. Having lost her quality of life, she chose to die a peaceful death with her family around her. It was a cathartic experience for all of us. We all miss her still.

Linda and I are about to embark on an extended road trip to Arizona and Southern California, starting with mountain biking with the F'n riders in Sedona. Linda's in Costa Rica right now. She left me to snowboard while she basked in sunshine and flowers. You can do that when you're retired.

This book is a worthy retirement project for me – promoting HPV cancer awareness, encouraging early throat cancer detection, and advocating for the immunization of boys. Boys are more prone to getting head and neck cancers from HPV, whereas girls, already have access to immunization, and are more likely to get cervical cancer from HPV. Given the response to my blog, I think other tongue cancer patients and their caregivers will take comfort and will gain insights from reading my story. Also, I can use the book to bring the world's attention to a lot of cancer and recovery causes. I'm up for that, and for whatever new adventures come with it.

Sharing my story, I'm reminded of just how privileged I am. Cancer is hard shit, but I had every advantage a person could have to survive it and recover. What if I hadn't been fit and healthy going in? I mightn't have come through as well. What if I'd still had to work and support a family? Many people do. I had the luxury of just being allowed to recover. What if I didn't have such a loving, supportive, and capable wife? Many people go through cancer alone. I can barely imagine how that would be. It would be so hard.

What if I weren't white, male, good-looking, athletic, educated, living in a city, living in a first world country, benefiting from universal health care, and blessed with the support of family and friends? I had all these advantages. Some earned, but most by accident of birth. Take any one of them away and cancer recovery would have been so much harder. Not everyone is so lucky. Most are not. I'm thankful to be so privileged.

That said, I still reserve some space for feeling sorry for myself. As my recovery extends into the rest of my life, I've become interested in what happens after treatment is over and the new normal has arrived. What I have endured, and what I now know is very common for cancer survivors, is an extended, low-grade depression. I have also suffered some serious losses. Losses that may never be recovered. I may never be as healthy and vibrant again. I'm still foggy-brained. Is that chemo brain, old age, or just the real me. It pervades every area of my life and I worry for myself. Linda worries too. Our relationship has changed and I worry that it'll never be the same. It's still good, but it used to be great.

The cancer community, those who treat people for cancer, recognizes that the cancer experience isn't over once you've been declared cancer free. For most survivors, there's a long period of adjustment to your new normal. A period that doesn't look challenging to outsiders, but it really is. That's what I'm going through now.

Having said that, I'm thankful to have a new normal to complain about.

The ride continues…just not quite as wild.

But next time it gets wild, I'll know how to handle it. There is no quit in me.

The End.

(There really is no 'end'. There is just carrying on, applying and passing on the lessons learned, one step at time, one after another, for as long as you've got)

TIME LINE FOR MY WILD RIDE WITH TONGUE CANCER

DISCOVERY:

OH SHIT, I HAVE CANCER!

First visits to the doctor for nasal problems	Jan and Feb 2016
Ultrasound - discovering I might have cancer	March 10, 2016
In very good shape, able to do 40 push ups, 4 pull ups, weight 165 lbs Snowboarding trip to Retallack with the Pow Crushers	March 11 - 15, 2016
CT Scan	March 17, 2016
Cancer diagnosis	March 18, 2016
First blog	March 22, 2016
PET Scan	March 24, 2016
Started feeling pains	March 27, 2016
Biopsy	April 5, 2016
Family gathering in Vancouver	April 16 and 17, 2016
Meeting with Gary Harvey	April 19, 2016
Meet with the Surgeon	April 22, 2016
Meet with Radiation and Chemotherapy oncologists	May 8, 2016
The Chinese Herbalist	May 16, 2016

TREATMENT:

I DIDN'T COME HERE TO LOSE.

First Chemo Treatment	May 24, 2016
First of 30 Radiation Treatments	May 25, 2016
X-rays taken of my swallowing	June 1, 2016
Fuck Cancer party	June 4, 2016
Sold the business, now retired	June 8, 2016

Second Chemo Treatment	June 14, 2016
Stopped eating – weight 136 lbs	June 18, 2016
Feeding tube inserted	June 21, 2016
Decide to not do 3rd round of chemo	June 28, 2106
Last Radiation Treatment	July 6, 2016

RECOVERY:
LET THE HEALING BEGIN

I quit talking	July 5 or so
Burns on my neck almost healed	July 20, 2016
Weight up to 149 lbs - 4 push-ups - no pull-ups	
Kayaking adventure	July 28, 2016
Started talking again	August 4, 2016
Scope shows no sign of the tumor	August 10, 2016
Started sipping water again	August 7, 2016
Eating a few sliced peaches	August 15, 2016
First slow bike ride after treatment	August 16, 1026
Road trip to Kamloops in Sprinter Van	End of August 2016
My first real meal - Won Ton soup	August 31, 2016

CANCER FREE:
I STILL FEEL LIKE SHIT

Trip to Winnipeg	Sept 19 to Oct 1, 2016
Facial pains from thrush	Early October, 2016
PET Scan – no tumor	Oct 18, 2016
Morphine reaction	October 27, 2016
Weight down to 136 lbs during thrush episode	
Thrush is gone	Early November, 2016

INTEGRATION:
NORMAL IS NOT WHAT IT USED TO BE

Swimming to get stronger   Early November 2016
First meeting with swallowing support group   Nov 10, 2016
CT Scan confirms cancer free   Nov 25, 2016
Feeding tube removed   Late November 2016
Weight 142 lbs and able to do 16 push-ups - 1 pull up
Snowboarding on river hills in Edmonton   Late December 2016
Surfing at a wave pool   Late December 2016
Learning to surf in Costa Rica   January and Feb 2017
Cat boarding trip to Retallack   March 12 -18, 2017
Mild PTSD diagnosis   April 2017
Retirement and Beat Cancer Party   May 12, 2017

MOVING ON

Back on my bike, but never the same   May 2017
New normal weight is 148 lbs - 24 push-ups, 2 pull ups
Sprinter Van trip to the west coast   June 2018
Moving on to a new life on Vancouver Island   September 2018

Note: this time line does not track my energy levels, degrees of pain, mucus flows, swallowing progress, changes in food tastes, chemo brain, sex drive or feelings of depression or optimism. For that you have to read the book.

Now, a year after moving to Vancouver Island, as of October 2018, the pains are gone. I still have some mucus and saliva problems and swallowing issues. I eat everything except spicy foods. My sex drive is back but diminished, and I am as optimistic as ever, riding my bike and snowboarding. I still weigh 148 pounds but I feel much stronger. No Quit in Me.

RESOURCES

MY GO-TO BOOKS FOR
MENTAL AND PHYSICAL HEALTH

Younger Next Year: Live Strong, Fit and Sexy – Until you're 80 and beyond
By Chris Crowley and Henry S. Lodge
Workman Publishing Company: New York, NY, 2007

The Emperor of All Maladies: A Biography of Cancer
By Siddhartha Mukherjee, an oncologist and researcher who won the 2011 Pulitzer Prize for this work.
Simon and Schuster: New York, NY, 2015

Flow: The Psychology of Optimal Experience
By Mihaly Csikszentmihalyi
Harper Perennial Modern Classics: New York, NY, 2008

Barbarian Days: A Surfing Life
By William Finnegan
Penguin Press: New York, NY, 2015

The Dwindling: A daughter's caregiving journey to the edge of life.
By Janet Dunnett
Journey's Press: Qualicum Beach, BC, 2017

Full Catastrophe Living: Using the Wisdom of Your Body and Mind to Face Stress, Pain and Illness (Revised Edition)
By Jon Kabat-Zinn
Bantam Books: New York, NY, 2013

SOME HELPFUL SITES

American Cancer Society
https://www.cancer.org/cancer/oral-cavity-and-oropharyn-geal-cancer.html

Canadian Cancer Society
http://www.cancer.ca/en/support-and-services/resources/publications/?region=on

The Oral Cancer Foundation
https://oralcancerfoundation.org

Support for People with Oral or Head and Neck Cancer (SPOHNC)
http://www.spohnc.org/

ACKNOWLEDGMENTS

This is a long list. There are more people to thank than I can name.

—

TO THE TEAM THAT HELPED PUT
THE BOOK AND WEBSITE TOGETHER.

Donaleen Saul who edited the blogs into a book. Donaleen Saul is an old friend of my wife, Linda, from their rabble-rousing years in their early 20s, and a veteran writer/editor. I appreciate her work in restructuring and editing my blogs so they flowed like a book, while preserving all the best parts and keeping my voice. I'm glad I trusted her.

JP King, book cover designer and interior layout artist. JP is Linda's daughter's husband. He's an artist and a publisher who has encouraged and advised me throughout the whole process. I appreciate his talent and professionalism.

Carol Sill, web designer, has given me good insight into how to market No Quit in Me and how to get the book into the hands of my intended readership, people affected by tongue cancer.

My son Michael Kuby for his revealing photo essay on my tongue cancer experience. See: www.michaelkuby.com

Dr. Brock Debenham and Anne Ryan's forewords were so well-written that I had to include them both.

My friends Peggy Arbeau and John Tansowny, as well as my sister Shenta Arnold, for their careful proof reading. Thanks for catching all those typos.

—

TO MY BLOG READERS:

I owe a debt of gratitude to my blog readers. The blog's success inspired this book. It had over 15,000 visits and over 1,000 comments.

—

TO THOSE WHO INSPIRED ME
TO TURN THE BLOG INTO A BOOK.

Faith Farthing is an editor who generously talked to me about what it takes to publish and market a book. Her faith in me kept the flame burning.

Janet Dunnett and Paul Shore are two local authors whose experience I drew on for publishing and marketing advice.

Ian Thornton, an intern at the Misericordia Hospital, who read my blog for most of the hour he was supposed to be shadowing my speech pathologist. He inspired me to turn the blog into a book.

—

TO THE DOCTORS, NURSES AND OTHER
MEDICAL STAFF WHO CARED FOR ME.

Dr. Brock Debenham, my radiation oncologist at the Cross Cancer Institute, who killed the cancer with radiation, was always cheerful and encouraging, and flattered me by calling me a high-functioning patient. He even came to the hospital on his day off to help me with a feeding tube issue that his intern could not handle.

Dr. John Walker, my chemotherapy oncologist, whose chemicals kicked the shit out of me but supported the radiation. He was always open and encouraging. He also introduced new patients to my blog.

Dr. Britteny Van Werkhoven, the locum doctor at the Links Clinic. She was just stepping in for my regular doctor, but she was quick to order an ultrasound test when my vague symptoms suggested that I might have cancer and concerned enough to give me her cell number so I could get the report from her quickly.

Dr. Glen Burchett, our family doctor, who had the job of telling Linda and I that I had tongue cancer. He described it as a particularly ugly cancer with potentially life changing effects. He assured us that I would likely survive but warned that it would be hard on both of us.

Dr. Jeffrey Harris, my surgical oncologist, who scared the shit out of us with his talk of surgically removing my whole tongue. That fear helped put my cancer journey into perspective.

Anna Sytsanko, my speech therapist, who helped me with my swallowing issues and who organized and facilitated the support group that Linda and I attended. I'm grateful for her patience and encouragement.

Patty Tachynski, my dietician, who had so many ideas for keeping my weight up and kept in touch with my progress long after treatment was over.

Karmen Schmidt, nurse practitioner in our tongue and throat cancer support group, who always offered helpful professional advice and an understanding perspective on what we were going through.

Dr. Jill Turner, the psychologist in our support group, for being there for us.

Oscar Mora, a nurse at the U of Alberta Hospital, with whom I bonded during my first PET scan. I promised to teach him snowboarding. I'm good for it.

Kyle, the guy who checked us in to the Cross Cancer Institute at every visit, and always laughed at my jokes.

The many nurses and technicians at the Cross Cancer institute, the University of Alberta Hospital, the Royal Alexandra Hospital, and the Misericordia Hospital. They were always cheerful and professional. I like that the nurses at the Cross always had me filling out questionnaires to monitor our changes. You asked about both health and psychological issues and even asked if we were experiencing financial difficulties. Impressive. Apparently, the doctors actually read them.

—

TO FELLOW TONGUE CANCER SUFFERERS WHO INSPIRED ME.

Dennis Richard, who was reading my blog before he met me in the support group and seemed genuinely appreciative of the information it provided. Dennis had surgery as well as radiation and chemo.

Franz Zabo, who was five months behind me in his treatment

and he and his wife found my blog to be useful as a way of tracking and predicting his progress

Al Slaney, a tongue cancer patient, who seemed to progress at the same pace as I did from radiation and chemotherapy. He'd been told by his surgeon that he probably had only ten months to live, that there was no treatment, and that he should "get his affairs in order." The radiation/chemo team took over his treatment and he recovered. Al filled the room at our support group meetings and was an inspiration. Sadly, Al has died recently from a completely different form of cancer.

Jan Prus-Czarnecki, an insightful contributor to our throat cancer support group who'd had cancer on his voice box, but after treatment that included surgery is speaking clearly and eating well.

Gary Warchola, who suffered through weeks of a strong burning sensation in his mouth after his radiation treatments. No one else in the group experienced that burning. An example of how each of us experiences cancer differently.

Scott Degen, who had surgery as well as radiation. He lost part of his tongue but did not seem impaired by it. I liked his sharing attitude in our support group.

—

TO MY FAMILY – FOR THEIR SUPPORT AND FOR THEIR MANY ACTS OF KINDNESS.

Linda Rasmussen, my loving wife. For enriching my life in so many ways, for being my tour guide to life, and for hanging in there with me when things got rough. As Elvis Presley said, "I love you for a hundred thousand reasons, but most of all I love you, because you're you."

Jeff Kuby, my son, for caring so deeply.

Michael Kuby, my son, for always being ready to talk with me, and for sharing my blog with others.

Kyle McCrea and Kirsten McCrea, Linda's son and daughter, who were always supportive and were insightful contributors to the blog.

Connie Mancheese, Jeff's long-time companion, who was always uplifting and who provided me with great book suggestions.

Danny, Dion, Rebecca, Kelley, Trevor and Katrina my nephews and nieces who tracked my progress and gaver me high fives.

Shenta Arnold, my sister, for always keeping in touch with me and for her wonderful Reiki treatments.

Gary Arnold, Shenta's husband and my friend, for his insights into the world of cancer.

D-Anne Kuby, my sister, for being present for me right from the start, for giving me permission to write as much as I wanted to, and for supporting me in having my own experience irrespective of others' advice.

Sandy Kuby, my brother, and his wife Rita, for their genuine concern and support.

Callie Kuby, for the "sound" advice that I didn't take and the healing thoughts.

Joyce Kuby, my late mother. After I did that whining in one of my blogs, she was quick to assure me that my father had loved me in his way. Always setting things right. She suffered a brain hemorrhage a year later at 96 and bravely chose a medically assisted death with the help of the M.A.I.D. Program. She was an inspiration to everyone who knew her. A much-loved woman.

Joyce Scott, Linda's mom, who followed my blog on her computer and who supported Linda, my main caregiver, by entertaining her with daily phone conversations.

Lorna Rasmussen, Linda's twin sister, and her husband George who always took time to support me.

Graydon McCrea, Linda's ex-husband, and his girlfriend Nan Schurmans, for caring and especially for bringing over a wonderful beef stew for Linda and me shortly after learning that I had cancer.

Freda Wapple, Linda's aunt, who expressed her concern and support through emails and the blog.

Dr. Glen Zenith, our dentist, married to Linda's cousin, for getting me in quickly to check for any necessary work on my teeth before my radiation started.

Margaret Langston, Linda's cousin, who really helped me with her "Hands of Light" treatments before and after my chemotherapy.

My son Michael's friends – Charli Elber, Steve Babish, Cayley Thomas Haug, Ily Barnes, Bryce Zimmerman and Ryan McFalls – for their concern for me.

—

TO MY PLAYGROUND AND RECREATION EQUIPMENT BUSINESS COMMUNITY.

The staff at PlayWorks and ParkWorks for taking care of business while I was ill, for being supportive, and for providing loyal service – Lori Vogelaar, Selena Madar, Jenny Harry, Debbie Souve, Pat Zelenak, Jay Silverman, Allie Perrin, Jacquie Lautermilch, Mitchell Taubensee, Melodie Ouellette, and Brian Davis.

Don Wong, my financial guy and loyal friend for over 35 years. He helped me build this business from a one-man gang to 15 full-time employees and $10M in sales during our better years.

Gerry, Garret and Kevin Vogelaar, Curtis Hrdlicka, Howard McIntyre, Lee Richard, Sheldon Tarry, who installed our playgrounds.

Pat Zelenak, the number one salesman at PlayWorks and all round "go to guy" for all things sales and project-related. A major contributor to my business success.

Jill White, who bought my business after I got sick. We couldn't have found a buyer more suited to making my company even better.

John Carvalho, who successfully and sensitively negotiated the sale of my business.

Ross Swanson, an excellent lawyer, who took care of the legal aspects of the business sale.

Serge Morin, a good friend and owner of Elephant Play, one of the playground companies we represented, who flew out from Montreal to Edmonton to be with Linda and me during radiation treatments.

Brad Friesen, a sales rep from Rubberstone, who took the time to come to our house for a visit after I sold the business.

Tisha Croome and Claude Vilgrain, two former PlayWorks sales reps, now friendly competitors, who reached out to me through the blog.

Brenda Field a former PlayWorks sales rep who sent her support.

Bev Wong, a former long-time employee, from 20 years ago, who contacted me from somewhere in the US, where she now lives with her husband and kids, to say she had been following the blog and that I'd been a mentor to her.

Margaret James and Dave Hilmer, both former employees and loyal friends from my days with Play and Learn who followed my progress.

My long-time friends from the Kompan, Inc. and BigToys, Inc. community over the last 35 years: Warren Baxter, Jeff Olson, Jay Beckwith, Tim Madely, Scott Ramsay, Susan Crawford, Valarie Wiggen, Natalie Haggen Child, Tom Grover, Tracy Themes, Bob Ross, Hap Parker, and David Parker.

Ben and Ruth Prins from Active Playgrounds, who sent me heartfelt, helpful, and caring emails and blog comments.

Pam Hoffman, Eric Von Dohlen and Denise Seidle from my days selling Romperland play equipment. Thank you for being there for me, then and now.

Kurt Krauss, the owner of Playcraft, one of our key manufacturers. Kurt was always a big supporter and a friend of Linda's and mine. Thanks Kurt for your faith in me and for support.

Dan Christensen from UPC parks – for the good banter.

TO THE F'N RIDERS
AND OTHER MOUNTAIN BIKING FRIENDS.

Andy Young, Tim Webber, Gerry Simpson, Nick Croken, Val Letawsky, Bryan Fontaine, Monika Mannke, and Kent Zucchet, who stopped by on their training rides to say hi and to have a beer. Ashley Ryniak, one of the Dirt Girls, who burned me a CD of tasteful folk, country and bluegrass music.

Val Letawsky, who loaned me a road bike when I couldn't mountain bike and Harry McKendrick, who introduced me to road biking on a long slow ride out in the country when I was ill.

Nick Croken, for taking some great photographs of me mountain biking in the river valley before I got too weak to ride.

Gary Ogletree for organizing the F'n riders and for continuing to keep me in the loop even when I was no longer riding with the group. And for making sure we all got those nice F'n Riders jerseys. I wore mine with pride when I went for my radiation treatments.

Gerry Ralph, an F'n Rider, for printing up the Fuck Cancer stickers and my noquitinme.com business cards.

Harvey Brauer, for always expressing an interest in me and my wellbeing and for the funniest and best comment on my blog. Steve Martins from Hard Core bikes, for getting me a stash of muscle-building fish oils from his wife Karen, another rider who is researching the effects of fish oil on cancer patients.

—

TO MY NEW BIKE RIDING BUDDIES
IN THE CUMBERLAND FOREST.

Gord Nettleton, Kelly Kostuik, Jay Nadler, Dave McDonald, Russ Thompson as well as Rocky Moise, all good guys and good riders who don't seem to mind if I slow them down a bit.

—

TO THE POW-POW CRUSHERS
(SKIERS AND SNOWBOARDERS).

A shout-out to those who were with me before I was diagnosed with tongue cancer, and remained in touch throughout my cancer adventure, especially to core members Joey Hundert, Tommy Kalita, James Knull, Ryan Kohen, and Jeff Fillmore, who were with me at last year's trip.
Chip Duffie, the Pow-Pow Crusher who coined the phrase "there is no quit in John Kuby" that inspired the title of my blog and now my book.

Antoine Palmer, organizer of the Pow-Pow Crushers, who is good enough to include me in the annual cat skiing/ snowboarding adventure, who took me out for some slow mountain biking while I was in treatment, and who, along with Chase Allen, introduced me to a first-class business broker to help me sell my business.

Jesse Hahn, a Pow-Pow Crusher, who took me to his yoga classes and took the time to connect for coffee and chats when I was ill.

Mike Geary, a Pow-Pow Crusher, who took the time to share some interesting video resources about cancer.

Marcus Gurske, who stayed in touch from Houston and shared his wife's cancer experience with me.

Pete Wardell, a Pow-Pow Crusher, who has kept in touch with me throughout this adventure – coming by to visit, taking me out for coffee, and sharing stories with me.

Ryan Brown, a Pow Crusher I always appreciated talking to. I was pleased when he became an avid bike rider and joined us on some of my healing rides as I recovered..

Thomas Beyer, a Pow-Pow Crusher, who offered banter and entertainment.

Ryan de Milliano, a Pow-Pow Crusher, who filmed and edited a YouTube video of me snowboarding, shortly after I found out I had cancer.

Judd de Val and Tommy Kalita for being there for me when I was coughing up blood after we left the bar the last night of our trip.

—

TO THE FRIENDS AND BLOG READERS
WHO SHARED THEIR THROAT CANCER
OR OTHER CANCER EXPERIENCES.

Gary Harvey, a TV director in Vancouver and an inspiring tongue cancer survivor, who generously gave of his time and attention throughout my cancer adventure.

Freda Van Niekerk, a friend of my mother's, who survived throat cancer a few years ago and is a bundle of positive energy.

When she heard about my situation, Freda contacted me and has been in touch ever since.

Lisa Reid-Branconnier, a fellow cancer patient whom I met at my first chemo treatment. She did the inspiring cancer doodle on page 105.

Mildred Thill, whom I knew first as a playground client and is now a friend, who had throat cancer as a child at a time when doctors knew less about treating it than they do now. An inspiring wisp of a woman with dynamite energy and a giving nature.

The surfer, snowboarder, and throat cancer survivor from Mexico and California whose email I have lost. I do remember his assuring me that I can still be a snowboarder and mountain biker after cancer.

Manon Aubry, whose cancer experience paralleled mine and who was generous with her advice and enthusiasm for my recovery.

Richard Stecenko, a cancer survivor, and his partner Lorna, who served a fabulous dinner for Linda and me in their charming home in Winnipeg, gave me hope that I would eventually say, "Oh yeah, I used to have cancer."

Judy, the yoga instructor at the Family Yoga Centre, also a cancer survivor, who assured me in a phone conversation that there was a lot to learn about myself from a cancer experience. She was right.

—

TO GOOD FRIENDS WITH WHOM WE HAVE BROKEN BREAD WITH OVER THE LAST WHILE.

Dave Gillespie and Karen Pumphrey, with whom we shared our first RV experience.

John Tansowny and his wife Peggy Arbeau, with whom we have broken bread several times since I was diagnosed. They always treated us like gold.

Dwayne Kushniruk and Gay, new friends who invited us over for a fabulous dinner early on in my cancer journey, and spent the evening watching John Kuby snowboard videos and listening to CDs of my favourite songs. It cheered me greatly.

Ernie and Beatrice Meili, old friends and business associates, who entertained us for a couple of days at their home in Candle Lake, Saskatchewan.

Kevin Taft and his wife Jeannette Boman, with whom we have shared dinners when I've been able to eat.

Catharine Phillips, a friend and former business coach, and her husband, Russ, for three enjoyable days at their summer home at East Barrier Lake near Kamloops in BC.

Phil Haug and Lorna Thomas for their thoughtful attention over the last year and for the delicious loaf Phil made. Lorna Thomas, a cancer survivor herself, continually touched base and offered good advice.

Deanne Morrow, one of Linda's long-time friends, who made me a beautiful blue quilt with bikes on it. I used it frequently throughout my treatment and recovery.

Brent Skidmore and Susan, friends in Lethbridge, who have stayed close to my situation through the blog and emails, and with whom we have shared meals.

—

TO OUR NEIGHBOURS IN RIVERDALE FOR THEIR MANY CONTRIBUTIONS.

James Rockey, who surprised me when I first told him I had tongue cancer by simply saying, "Ya, it'll be tough, but you'll get over it." Turns out he was right.

Paul and Monica Iglinsky, neighbours, who inspire Linda and me every time we see them going out for one of their long walks.

Rocky Feroe, who calls me the Kubinator the Cancernator. She also told me after I had lost 25 pounds that I was still good-looking.

Jeremy Baumung, all-round good guy, accomplished actor and an apprentice electrician, who did a bunch of electrical work for us. Rob and Zane who inspire us with their wholesomeness and industrious home owner activity.

Kris Currier and his girlfriend as well as Scott Zucchet, who joined us for our little "fuck cancer" party one July weekend. I enjoyed the mountain bike ride we went on.

—

TO MY MANY MEMORABLE BLOG COMMENTERS.

Brent Skidmore, a friend from high school with a shared spirit of adventure. He is a prolific writer who has had more health issues than the average person. His comments came from that depth of experience.

Patty Burke, a friend from my 20's. Patty has had cancer twice and has lost loved ones to cancer, so her caring, insight, and steady stream of wisdom came from a place of having lived with cancer.

Aina O'Malley, a friend of Patty's, also a cancer survivor. When I was about 20 years old Aina turned me on to reading books and changed my life forever.

Greg Matthes, one of my best friends, who lives on a sailboat on the west coast with his wife Kris. Greg only commented twice on the blog but charmed me each time.

Cole Summers, a friend since high school, who has been a personal trainer for 45 years. He reminded me that we all become like the five or six people we hang out with. I try to hang out with people who strive to be fit, well-informed and principled, like Cole.

Kerry Suche, long-time friend and confidante with whom I first explored "how to be an effective salesman" over 40 years ago.

Will Lawrence, a friend from university and former business partner, who surprised me by telling me in a blog comment that he had once had cancer. Who knew?

Ken Friesen for his description of watching me skate as a teenager and admiring how fluid it was. I think he compared me to Gretzky, but Gretzky was not even born then.

David Wager, a friend from university, whose one comment was, "It is ironic that the man with the golden tongue would get throat cancer."

Lori Webber, wife of an F'n rider, whose supportive comments meant a lot since she is living bravely through a chronic health issue that is much worse than what I was dealing with.

Kristin Gardiner, good friend, regular reader, frequent commenter, and always a cheerleader.

Marg Artis, a valuable employee in the formative years of my company, a regular reader and loyal friend.

Val (Watt) Goodridge, a high school friend and cancer survivor, who frequently had something encouraging and supportive to add.

Jim French and his wife Val, from Silver Heights Collegiate days in Winnipeg, who have followed my blog from day one and provided attentive comments.

Joan Arnold, for always paying attention and offering cheerful encouragement.

Kent Zucchet, almost always the first to respond to a new post. Cheryl Caul, a nurse practitioner, who always had our backs if the medical community got it wrong.

Sandra Stuart, a friend and yoga instructor in Winnipeg for caring about me and for giving me breathing exercises.

Jeff Olson, from my BigToys days, 20 years ago. He not only followed the blog and commented, but he made me a member of his adventure junkie group called HARD (Horny, Ancient, Radical Dudes). He even mailed me a HARD t-shirt.

Brenan Prins, who contributed and sent me emails that offered prayers and testimonials to the power of faith.

To the many blog readers from faith-based communities, who included me in their prayers. I may not believe in God, but I have faith in the power of prayer.

—

There are bound to be friends and associates whom I have forgotten to acknowledge. I am thankful, but I am often also forgetful. May I be forgiven.

Dear Reader,

If you think No Quit in Me has value, then please ask yourself, "Who should know about this book?"

If anyone you know is being touched by cancer and you think they would find good companionship in "No Quit in Me", then please gift them a copy, share a link to our website www.noquitinme.ca, and post a review on Amazon. Please help others find this book.

Thank you for being a "No Quitter" and helping others to become "No Quitters" too.

- John Kuby

Stay tuned to the website for news, events, and more:

www.noquitinme.ca

- Follow the blog and set alerts for new posts
- Sign up for the email list
- Check out the photo essay: www.michaelkuby.com
- Order books, t-shirts, mugs, and more!

On Facebook – "No Quit in Me Book"

- Follow my progress and the book's progress
- Discover book promotions, speaking engagements, and event notices
- Give us your feedback